OXFORD M

Kidney Failure

THE FACTS

Kidney Failure

THE FACTS

STEWART CAMERON

Emeritus Professor of Renal Medicine
Guy's–St. Thomas' Hospitals
London

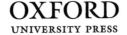

OXFORD
UNIVERSITY PRESS

OXFORD

UNIVERSITY PRESS

Great Clarendon Street, Oxford OX2 6DP

Oxford University Press is a department of the University of Oxford.
It furthers the University's objective of excellence in research, scholarship,
and education by publishing worldwide in

Oxford New York

Auckland Bangkok Buenos Aires Cape Town Chennai
Dar es Salaam Delhi Hong Kong Istanbul Karachi Kolkata
Kuala Lumpur Madrid Melbourne Mexico City Mumbai Nairobi
São Paulo Shanghai Singapore Taipei Tokyo Toronto

and an associated company in Berlin

Oxford is a registered trade mark of Oxford University Press
in the UK and in certain other countries

Published in the United States
by Oxford University Press Inc., New York

First published 1996
Reprinted 1998 (twice), 1999, 2002

A catalogue record for this book is available from the British Library

Library of Congress Cataloging in Publication Data
Cameron, J. Stewart (John Stewart)
Kidney failure / Stewart Cameron.
(The facts)
Includes index
1. Chronic renal failure. I. Title. II. Series: Facts (Oxford,
England)
RC918.R4C35 1996 616.6'14—dc20 96–8019
ISBN 0 19 262643 4

Printed in Great Britain by
Biddles Ltd, Guildford and King's Lynn

What is man, when you come to think upon him, but a minutely set, ingenious machine for turning, with infinite artfulness, the red wine of Shiraz into urine. You may even ask which is the more intense craving and pleasure: to drink, or to make urine?

Karen Blixen (Isak Dinesen): *Dreamers*,
Seven Gothic Tales, p. 233. Panther/Triad Books,
London and St Albans

Foreword

This book follows on from its predecessor, *Kidney disease—the facts*, but concentrates on kidney failure. It does not aim to cover common kidney conditions such as urinary tract infections and cystitis which do not cause kidney failure; or forms of nephritis (Bright's disease) which do not go on to cause kidney failure.

Focusing on kidney failure allows me to go into more detail on the causes, and especially the treatment of this unfortunate condition. Here we deal with what you can expect from the moment you or a relative or friend is told they have a degree of kidney failure, through to when treatment is begun, and what continuing the treatment will be like. Naturally many worries and topics to think about come up when you learn you have kidney failure: how you will feel, your job, your family, your independence, and concern about the future. I hope this book will give some information which, together with information from the team of doctors, nurses, counsellors, and social workers who are looking after you, will help you cope better with the problems you face. I have tried to be completely honest throughout this book: if a treatment does not exist, I have said so; if problems are likely to arise, I have listed them.

As with its predecessor, this book is dedicated to all those patients with kidney failure whom I have been privileged to help look after during the past 35 years, and from whom I have learned all that I know. This book is to a great extent the sum of their experiences.

London   J.S.C.
July 1996

Contents

Introduction

Kidney failure is not by any means the commonest cause of death or disability. In Britain, while 250 000 people die each year of heart and blood vessel diseases, and more than 150 000 from cancers, only 7000 go into kidney failure. The figures for heart and blood vessel disease and cancers in the United States are proportionately almost exactly the same, only four times greater because of the much bigger population, although the numbers going into end-stage kidney failure are bigger in proportion (about 75 000 each year) because kidney failure is more common. Why then should we bother with such a rare condition?

Although we cannot prevent the majority of people developing end-stage kidney failure, we can treat them successfully by replacing their kidney function. Most people know that there are two major ways in which this can be done: either to use a kidney machine to do the work of the now failed kidneys, or to have a kidney transplant. Both are generally successful, although each treatment has its problems which we will discuss later in this book. Currently 25 000 Britons and 200 000 Americans receive treatment for kidney failure, and worldwide almost a million people owe their lives to this form of therapy. Each year the number increases.

For each patient, treatment for kidney failure is *very* expensive, although other treatments which are even more expensive are coming into use each year. The UK spends about £300 million each year—and needs to spend much more—whilst the United States spends a staggering 7 billion dollars every year on the treatment of end-stage kidney failure. Thus both the public and governments have been aware of the difficult issues raised by the success and the high costs of treatments for end-stage kidney disease.

Kidney failure becomes more common with increasing age. Thus of the 7000 people going into kidney failure each year in the UK, about 2000 are over 80 years of age, and 5000 are over 50. What should be done for the very elderly person with kidney failure is now a major problem in all developed countries, and issues of when treatment should be given or withheld have engaged the attention not only of the public and governments, but also of ethicists, sociologists, and religious leaders. When a very elderly individual is treated for kidney failure and later becomes demented or otherwise damaged, can one, should one withdraw treatment; and on what grounds, and how and who should decide?

Wider issues arise also in connection with transplantation, the most successful way of replacing renal function. Everywhere in the world there is a relative shortage of donor kidneys from the recently dead, and waiting lists for kidney transplants become longer and longer every year. A kidney from a close relative is probably the most successful treatment of all, but raises problems of whether someone who is fit and well should have an 'unnecessary' operation— so far as they are concerned—which carries some risk. Finally a major problem in many Third World countries is the problem of people, almost always poor, or convicted prisoners, being paid or coerced to give a kidney to someone who needs it. This, in world terms, is the major form of transplantation, and raises even more complex issues, even though this form of transplantation is banned by law in almost all developed countries, and in many developing countries as well. Much attention has been paid to the possibility of using animal kidneys, such as from pigs or baboons, but we need much more research before we know if this will prove feasible.

The moment you find out that you, or a close relative, partner, or friend, have kidney failure is a bewildering and frightening time. For some the worry is that the kidney problem will progress to kidney failure, and what can be done to prevent or slow this, and what all the confusing tests and their results mean. Others, less fortunate, are already in kidney failure and facing the imminent need to start dialysis (kidney machine or similar treatment). Then there is a bewildering choice of possible courses. Everyone seems to speak a strange jargon, half familiar and half difficult or impossible to understand. This book is designed to help you understand what may be going on. You may choose, if (for example) you are already starting on CAPD treatment, to turn straight to Chapter 7 to see what there is today about this treatment. Others will be most in need of advice about progressing kidney disease and will need to concentrate on Chapters 3 or 4. However, before we consider kidney *failure*, it's worth looking briefly at what kidneys do in health, why we need them, and what is likely to go wrong if they fail.

1 *What do kidneys do?*

What am I, life? A thing of watery salt
Held in cohesion by unresting cells
Which work they know not why, which never halt
Myself unwitting where their master dwells

John Masefield: *Sonnets*, No. 37, 1910.

It is no exaggeration to say that the composition of the blood is determined, not by what the mouth takes in, but by what the kidneys keep.

Homer W. Smith: *From Fish to Philosopher*, Chapter 1. Little Brown, Boston (1955).

To understand better what goes wrong when kidneys fail to function, it's worth knowing a little about what they do in health, and their role in maintaining a healthy state of well-being. If you are a patient, or a patient's relative, who is already in kidney failure and facing the prospect of dialysis or transplantation, you may prefer to skip to the chapters which deal with the particular disease you suffer from (Chapters 3 and 4), what happens in kidney failure (Chapter 5), or to those on dialysis (Chapters 6 and 7), or after transplantation (Chapter 8).

Most people, if asked the question 'What do kidneys do?' would answer: 'Make urine, of course'. This answer begs the question, since next we have to ask: 'What is urine'? and even more important: '*Why* urine'? Why do we need kidneys at all? Why do we die if they stop functioning?

Why do we have kidneys?

Complex living things such as human beings are made up of many, many individual *cells*—about 10^{15} cells, that is a thousand million million individual living units. These cells are organized into *tissues* such as fat, muscle, blood, or the system which protect us against invaders such as bacteria (germs) and viruses; and *organs* such as the heart, liver, brain, lung, or kidney. Many organs are predominantly made up of one sort of cell, but almost all organs have in them at least a small number of different types of cells and tissues.

Only 500 or 600 million years ago a number of cells associated together to form *many-celled organisms*, of which we are an example. The advantages of this were the ability to enter newer, even harsher environments and exploit them to stay alive. This gathering together of a number of cells requires a number of extra features: first, an outer coat to keep the thing together; secondly, as the organism increases in size, a means of circulating substances needed to keep the cells going (for example, glucose and oxygen) and a means of removing their products (e.g. carbon dioxide): in short, a circulation, and with it eventually as organisms became larger, something to pump the fluid around—a heart.

What do kidneys do?

If the many-celled organism is to roam widely, it must carry within its outer coat, but outside the cells themselves, a second 'soup' which allows the transport of the fuels and wastes into and out of the cells. The idea of this 'extracellular fluid' was first conceived a century and half ago, and the principal task of the kidney is to *preserve the volume and the composition of this extracellular fluid constant* (Figure 1).

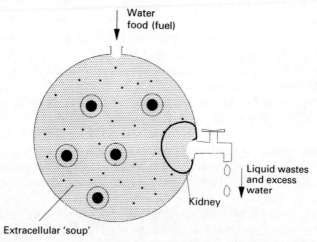

Figure 1   The role of the kidneys in regulating the volume and composition of the body's extracellular 'soup'. The cells (small circles with dark centres) are bathed in a fluid which provides them with an environment in which they function well, and which is contained within the outer skin of the organism. The kidney's main function is to maintain constant the composition and volume of this extracellular 'soup'.

A part of this task—but only a part—is to rid the body of some of the waste products of the cells' activities (metabolism) which the cells cannot break down further. Thus the principal function of the kidney is *not excretion, but regulation.*

We can move and survive on dry land, even though three-quarters of us is water, our cells tucked away in a carefully guarded cradle of extracellular fluid, whose composition is preserved with exquisite accuracy by our kidneys, a major part of our life-support system in this hostile environment. We can roam into deserts, and (usually) survive, or drink six pints of beer, or starve, or gorge, but essentially the extracellular 'soup' bathing our cells remains constant in quality and quantity, and because of this, the composition of the cells themselves is kept constant. The kidney has less control of what goes on inside the cells, since given that the kidneys do their job adequately, each cell is to a large extent autonomous, and will extract and eject what it needs or does not need from the extracellular fluid.

The kidney obviously conserves what we need, but even more it permits us *the freedom of excess.* That is, it allows us to take in more than we need of many necessities—water and salt for example—and excretes exactly what is not required. This is essential since neither we nor our ancestors know or knew the composition of the foods we eat, and the only way to ensure a sufficiency of everything is to eat an excess of at least some things.

Finally, the kidneys preserve the *volume* of our body fluids as well as their composition. Given that we are almost three-quarters water, the precision with which the kidney achieves this can be assessed quite simply by weighing oneself each day. Despite variations in diet, exercise, or fluid intake, the figures remain constant, sometimes depressingly so! This illustrates how precisely the kidney performs its tasks, with a precision of as good as 1 per cent and never worse than 5 per cent, under very varying circumstances.

Therefore, if your kidneys fail right now, suddenly, you will die only after perhaps a week, in part because some of the accumulated waste-products of metabolism are toxic to the heart, which stops. More complicated and important is the way in which the kidney can *adapt* to slow destruction by disease, so that one can survive on as little as 5 per cent of overall kidney function, or (if the kidney's job is minimized by careful adjustments of input) down to even 3 per cent. The advantages of this gift of 20 times more kidney than we need to survive are not obvious, except to allow a wide margin of excess, since well before this point you cannot function normally, even in a civilized environment, but the kidney has enormously greater reserve capacity in the face of disease than (for example) the heart or the lungs.

What are kidneys like and how do they function?

The kidneys are a pair of organs which are situated towards the back of the body, just at the level of the waist (Figure 2). Each lies in a small pad of fat, on the muscles at the back of the abdomen. The upper part of the kidney lies under the ribs, so that the kidneys are protected from damage to some extent. They receive their blood supply from the main artery of the body, the aorta, and give blood back to the main vein, the vena cava. Each kidney is about 10–15 cm (about 5 inches) long, and weighs about 160 g (6 oz). From each kidney, urine is conducted in two tubes, the ureters, which join the bladder, which is down in the pelvis. The bladder is a hollow muscular bag, which can expand to contain urine and store it before it is passed. The average capacity of an adult bladder is about 500–750 ml (a pint, or a pint and a half) before you feel uncomfortable and need to pass urine.

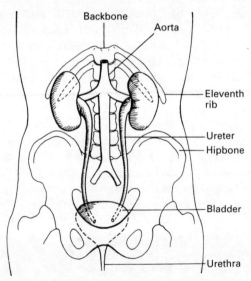

Figure 2   The position of the kidneys. From the kidneys, the ureters conduct urine to the bladder, and hence through the urethra. Blood is supplied by two renal arteries from the aorta, the main artery of the body.

Each kidney is not a single organ, but is made up of about one million units, called *nephrons* (from the Greek word for kidney, *nephros*). The Latin word is *renes*, so that you will meet a number of words containing the roots nephr- (e.g. nephron, nephrology unit, nephrologist) and ren- (e.g. renal clinic). Each

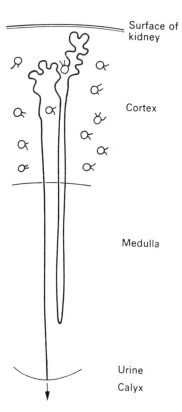

Figure 3 Diagram of a single unit of the kidney, the *nephron*. Each kidney is made up of approximately one million nephrons. The glomerular filter is near the surface of the kidney, supplied by blood. The tubular fluid is gradually modified into urine by the long tubule, which loops down into the medulla, then back again into the cortex, then back into the medulla again. This arrangement allows greater length for the tubule, and this also allows the urine to be concentrated (see text).

of these nephron units is to some extent autonomous, but it would be a mistake to regard kidney function as merely the sum of the action of two million nephrons. The architecture of the kidney allows the whole to do more than the sum of its parts could do.

Each nephron (Figure 3) consists of two parts: a filter (called the *glomerulus*) and a *tubule* leading out from it. The glomerulus (Figure 4) is a bunch or tuft of blood capillaries (the smallest vessels of the circulation) with especially thin

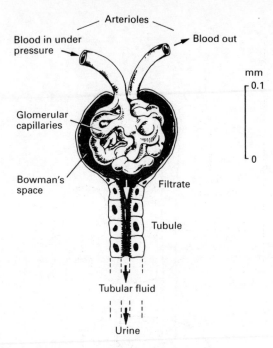

Figure 4 A single glomerulus, magnified about 400 times. Blood comes into the glomerular filter by the small artery (arteriole) at the top left, and passes through the cluster of very small blood vessels (capillaries) which make up the glomerular tuft, leaving via the outgoing (efferent) arteriole at the top right. Using the pressure generated by the heart's contractions, fluid is forced through into the space around the glomerulus, named Bowman's space after the first person to describe the glomerulus accurately. This filtrate then enters the tubule, where the cells lining it progressively modify the filtrate into urine, greatly reducing it in volume during the process.

walls to permit it to act as a filter. The glomeruli can just be seen as tiny red dots in the cut surface of a fresh kidney, more easily visible under a magnifying glass. Under the microscope, the tuft resembles a raspberry, with the small blood vessels entering and leaving at the 'stalk'. The tubules drain the filtered fluid from the glomerulus, but are not straight. They loop downwards, and since the glomeruli lie in the outer part of the kidney (the rind, or *cortex*) which contains both glomeruli and tubules (Figure 5), while there is an inner part which contains no glomeruli, but only tubules. This is called the *medulla* (Figure 5). If you take a pork, mutton, or beef kidney from the butcher's and cut it open, these two layers, the cortex and the medulla, can be distinguished clearly: the darker outer cortex and the inner lighter-coloured medulla. The

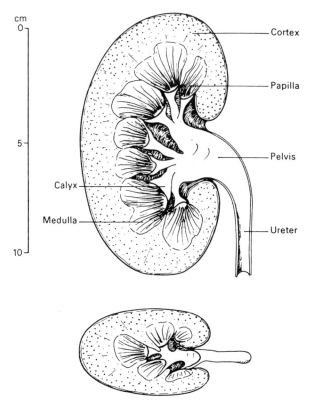

Figure 5　A kidney cut lengthwise and across. The outer layer, the *cortex*, is stippled
to indicate that the glomerular filters present within it are just visible to the naked eye,
whilst the inner *medulla* appears striped, because the tubules run in parallel through it.
Each subdivision of the medulla ends in a *papilla*, which discharges urine into the
calyces. These form the pelvis of the kidney, which narrows down to form the ureter.
　　The calyces and pelvis are surrounded by fat (dark in the diagram).

cortex contains glomerular filters and tubules; the medulla contains the tubules
only. These as we have just noted, do not drain directly but first loop inward
into the medulla and then pass back into the cortex to enter the medulla again
(Figure 3). Human kidneys resemble pork kidneys more than the others, since
beef and mutton kidney are lumpy (lobulated) in a way human and pig kidneys
are not. In fact human kidneys are shaped very much like kidney beans.

　　The blood supply of the kidneys enters at the centre and fans out into smaller
and smaller vessels, most of the blood going to perfuse the cortex and its

glomeruli for filtration of fluid from it. The veins return into bigger and bigger vessels, reversing the fan, and the main renal vein comes out beside the renal artery going in. The urine emerging from the individual nephrons is collected into about five or six cup-shaped collection tracts (calyces) which join to form a bag which lies partly outside the substance of the kidney (confusingly called the pelvis, like the bony pelvis into which our legs fit). This pelvis of the kidney lies beside the artery and vein, and leads into the ureter, which conducts urine to the bladder for storage before it is passed into the outside world.

How do kidneys work?

Each glomerulus takes in blood under pressure and filters off about one fifth of the water in that blood together with its dissolved salts. However it lets through no cells and virtually no larger molecules such as proteins. This is important in the diagnosis of kidney disease, because in normal urine there is virtually no protein and no cells. In diseases affecting the glomeruli however, both cells and proteins and even some unaltered blood can pass into the urine and can be tested for in the urine (see Chapter 2). The volume of filtered fluid formed is very large—for the two kidneys it is about 200 litres (50 gallons) every 24 hours! A moment's thought reminds us that the body only contains, on average, about 50 litres (12 gallons) of water, so that your kidneys *recycle all the water in your body four times a day.*

Clearly, nearly all of this filtered water and salts must be retrieved, and in fact about 99.5 per cent of salt and water are normally reabsorbed in the tubule, so that only about 1.5–2.5 litres (3–5 pints) of urine are finally passed each day, as everyone knows. Thus, in the next step the tubule transforms the filtrate into urine, whilst reducing it greatly in volume. Why on earth do we have a kidney which throws away far more than we could ever afford, and then grabs almost all of it back again?

Our problem, on dry land, is finding and conserving water. However this has only been a problem for about 100 million years. The problem of a fish living in fresh or brackish water is quite different. All the time, he (or she) is being assaulted in the tendency of water to *enter* the body, since the extra-cellular fluid has a greater concentration of salts than the surrounding water. The obvious answer is to evolve a pressure-filter kidney which can get rid of large volumes of water easily. But what if this 'fish' spends more and more time lounging around on sandbanks gulping air, like the mud-skipper does today? It must start retrieving some of that water which now becomes valuable. Possibly this is how we came to have our two-stage glomerulus-tubule kidney. Even so, doing it this way does have its advantages. The kidney must do some very fine tuning of the body fluids as we have seen, and one way of doing this very accurately is to do a small amount of work on a very large volume, monitoring all the time what is going on.

One of the most important jobs the tubules perform, besides determining the amount of water in the body, is to regulate the amount of salt (sodium and chloride) which is excreted. Just as with water, much more salt than the body contains is filtered each day through the glomeruli. The great bulk of salt is reabsorbed—99 to 99.5 per cent—and the exact amount must be regulated to match exactly the output needed to maintain the body's salt normal and constant. Thus, by and large input will match output to input in health. Output can vary from 0.5 to 15 g (one twentieth to half an ounce) of salt per day, a thirty-fold variation. Day in, day out, the kidney achieves this almost to perfection, but the exact mechanisms which regulate sodium absorption in the tubules still eludes us despite many decades of research. Much of this control is achieved within the kidney, the rest by response to chemical messengers, usually called hormones, after the Greek for messenger: this is discussed later.

The kidney tubules normally reabsorb some other dissolved substances completely, such as glucose, and amino acids (the building bricks of protein) since these are valuable. Why do we first filter these, and then reabsorb them? The reason is that the glomerular filter cannot be set to keep these in, and also permit some substances of the same size such as uric acid, urea, and creatinine which are all end-products of the body's metabolism, and like ash from a fire, to be cleared away if the fire is not to go out. The kidney, in fact, does not get this one quite right, because some urea, and most of the uric acid are re-absorbed and have to be re-excreted again, whilst all the creatinine is got rid of. The urea is used to help in the mechanism which determines how concentrated the urine is, i.e. how much water is excreted, but reabsorbing uric acid is simply a nuisance, making us liable to gout.

The mechanism of determining how much water is excreted is complicated, and depends upon the arrangement of tubules as long loops, with loops of blood vessels following. This allows the medulla of the kidney to accumulate a higher concentration of dissolved substances than anywhere else in the body. This high concentration around the tubules can be used in turn to allow the formation of urine of high concentration, with the extraction of most of the water as the final stage of urine information.

The kidney tubule also has an important function in ridding the body of excess acid (hydrogen ions). It does this both by secreting them direct from the blood into the filtrate, and also in the form of ammonium which contains one hydrogen ion. (The ammoniacal smell or urine, however, arises from the breakdown of urea to ammonium, and not from the tiny amount excreted as such.)

A final point needs consideration, and that is why we have to pass urine all the time. Why can't we switch off urine production altogether in times of drought? This is impossible because of two constraints. The first is that there is an upper limit to the concentration of urine that we can achieve. This is a function of the length of the loops in the kidney tubules—animals such as hamsters and gerbils, which can excrete urine from two to five times more concentrated than we, have much longer tubules, and need to have a kidney medulla which hangs right down the ureter to accommodate them. The other constraint, given that there is a limit to our concentrating capacity, is that there is a minimum amount of soluble waste which we *must* excrete through our kidneys each day. This is mostly nitrogen-containing compounds, principally urea; and on a normal diet we produce an amount which will not dissolve in less than about 500–600 ml (one pint) of the most concentrated urine we can produce. Therefore, even on a raft in the Pacific, or in the Sahara we go on passing this volume of urine, whether we like it or not. Incidentally, this tells you why it's fatal to drink your urine under these circumstances—it's already four times as concentrated as your blood, if you are dehydrated.

These unhappy results are a consequence of our ancestors having 'chosen' urea as the end-product for our metabolism of nitrogen-containing compounds. Birds, snakes, lizards, and spiders have chosen uric acid, which is insoluble, and can be dropped as a slurry with almost no water—as anyone who has stood under a treeful of starlings at dusk can testify. This makes them better at surviving in dry environments.

What controls kidney function?

So far I have talked about the kidney as though it operated entirely on its own in response to changes in the composition of the body fluids. Nothing could be further from the truth. Although the kidney is the final arbiter, it needs information fed to it from elsewhere in the body to tell it what to do (Figure 6).

Some of this information is sensed *directly* by the kidney, first by looking at the stretch of the small arteries going into each glomerular filter; secondly, by monitoring the composition of the filtered fluid within the tubule. These two mechanisms within the kidney itself give it a good baseline for both the blood pressure within the circulation, and the sodium in the filtrate—and hence the blood.

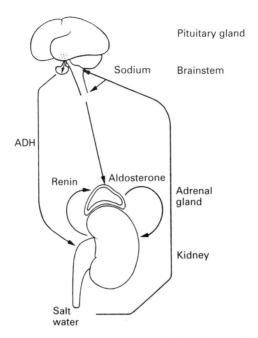

Figure 6 Control of the kidney's management of salt and water. This consists of a series of 'feedback loops', involving the kidney itself, the brain and its associated pituitary gland, blood vessels within and without the kidney, and the adrenal gland (see text). Between them the volume and composition of the body's fluids is managed with exquisite accuracy.

However, there are other mechanisms outside the kidney which send messengers (hormones) to the kidney (Figure 6). The first of these is the mechanism in the brain which senses the overall concentration of dissolved substances in the blood, and sends a hormone (antidiuretic hormone, ADH) to modulate the final amount of water which is extracted in final formation of the urine. The higher the blood concentration, the more ADH is secreted and the more water is reabsorbed, so that less urine is passed. The effects of some familiar substances occur through this pathway: alcohol—even when taken without a lot of water, in the form of 'shorts'—switches off ADH and the resultant inappropriate increase in urine volume depletes the body of water. Dehydration forms part of a hangover, and a couple of glasses of water before going to bed will usually improve how you feel. Conversely, nicotine in cigarettes inhibits ADH production and urine volume, all other things being equal, will fall.

The second mechanism is more complicated and determines how much salt the kidney excretes, which in turn determines the overall volume of the extra-cellular fluid. 'Volume receptors' within the circulation, especially the veins entering the heart, prompt the production of a hormone called atriopeptin, or ANP, which acts directly on the kidney to promote less of sodium; and another, from the central nervous system, stimulates the adrenal gland just above each kidney to produce a second hormone (aldosterone), which promotes retention of sodium in the tubule.

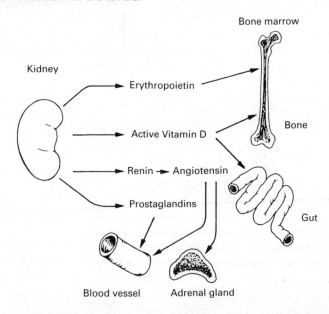

Figure 7 The kidney's hormones. Four main hormones (or groups of hormones in the case of the prostaglandins) are produced, which act on the different organs indicated in the diagram. ADH stands for antidiuretic hormone (see the text).

The kidney as a hormone producer (Figure 7)

So far we have concentrated upon the obvious functions of the kidney: regulation and excretion. Now we have to finish this chapter by considering a third important function: the *secretion* of hormones, or messengers which tell other cells in the body what to do. We don't think of the kidney as a gland, but in fact like most organs in the body it produces hormones as well as responding to them.

Renin

The first of these hormones which the kidney produces is called, appropriately, *renin*. This is part of one of the regulatory mechanism of salt and water, and is produced by cells just beside each glomerulus apparatus. Renin of itself has no action, but it acts on a protein in the bloodstream to produce a small molecule, which is then acted on by a second protein, which leads to a final product with very powerful effects: *angiotensin*. First, it constricts blood vessels and raises the blood pressure, which is important in high blood pressure and in its treatment (see Chapter 4), and one can predict that people with kidney trouble might under some circumstances get high blood pressure; this is of course the case. Secondly, it stimulates the kidney to retain sodium; and thirdly, it stimulates the adrenal gland to produce the hormone mentioned above, aldosterone, which is triggered by volume receptors within the circulation.

Vitamin D

It may come as a surprise to learn that the second hormone which the kidney produces is the active form of *vitamin D*. This vitamin is essential for the formation and maintenance of healthy bone, and promotes the absorption of calcium from the gut. Being a vitamin it is a compound that we must have in our diet because we cannot make it ourselves. Without it, children get the bone disease *rickets*, adults the similar disease of bones which have finished growing, called *osteomalacia* (soft bones). However, before vitamin D can act on bone or on calcium absorption it must be transformed twice, first in the liver, and then in the kidney to its active form. One could predict from this that patients with kidney disease might suffer from bone problems, and this is indeed the case.

Erythropoietin (EPO)

Third, the kidney produces a hormone which promotes the formation of red blood cells by the bone marrow. Red blood cells are called erythrocytes in Greek, and the hormone is called *erythropoietin*. It is released from the kidney if the oxygen in the blood falls low, for example, on going to high altitudes. Again one could predict that patients without kidneys or with kidney disease would become anaemic; and this is indeed the case, although EPO deficiency is not the entire story.

Prostaglandins

Finally, the kidney produces several of an important group of compounds, the *prostaglandins*. As their name suggests, these substances were first identified in secretions from the prostate gland in men. Some are very important in regulating blood-flow, sodium excretion, and blood pressure and are produced in the kidney. Probably they are part of the kidney's own regulation of its blood-flow.

Summary

Thus the kidney regulates the composition and volume of the fluid bathing the cells of the body, excretes waste end-products of the body's chemical factories, and makes a number of important messengers which have effects outside as well as within the kidney. Thus when kidneys fail, all three of these important functions will be compromised.

2 *How will I know if I have kidney disease?*

When the patient dies the kidneys may go to the pathologist, but while he lives the urine is ours. It can provide us day by day, month by month, and year by year with a serial story of the major events going on within the kidney. The examination of the urine is the most essential part of the physical examination of any patient with Bright's disease.

Thomas Addis: *Glomerular nephritis, diagnosis and treatment*. Chapter 1. Macmillan, New York (1948).

Symptoms and signs of kidney disease

How will I know if I have kidney disease?

The answer to this question is that you may very well *not* know. Kidneys are not very demonstrative organs, even when seriously in trouble. Part of the reason for this is the huge excess of kidney function which we have for normal circumstances. You can survive fairly comfortably on only 10% of normal kidney function, although an observant person will realize that some things are wrong. Thus kidney disease is often picked up on testing the urine as a routine part of some other examination, or because a blood test is done, again for some other reason, and the test indicates that the kidneys are in trouble.

In the next couple of chapters we will go on to consider specific kidney diseases which can cause kidney failure, but here we will look at the ways in which kidney trouble may come to your attention. After all, it's not disease that you complain of, it's what your doctor calls *symptoms*, that is, things you notice. By convention, *signs* are what the doctor finds on examination, either physical examination of the body, or on chemical, radiological, or other examination, such as special tests.

Normally there are no outward signs of kidney function except the fact that you pass urine from time to time. There is no way of reminding yourself that your kidneys are working from moment to moment, such as feeling the pulse, counting respirations, or performing a knee jerk. Also, many patients with quite severe kidney failure may have no specific complaints, or only mild feelings which may be dismissed as just being tired; this point is discussed further in Chapter 5. In fact, those patients who have a lot of symptoms from their kidneys are often those with the mildest and least serious conditions, which do not go on to damage the kidney permanently.

Urine

It's easy to forget just what a remarkable substance urine is. In ancient and medieval times it was used as a resource, since it contains valuable nitrogen and phosphate in considerable amounts. The Roman emperor Vespasian passed laws governing the collection of urine from public urinals, and the now rapidly vanishing *pissoirs* of Paris, and other French and Italian cities, are still named after him (Vespasiani). It was also used on the crofts of the Outer Hebrides to prepare and shrink Harris tweed, since aged urine contains ammonia—which accounts perhaps for the peculiar smell of a genuine Harris tweed when wet. Finally, being warm and (normally) sterile when first passed, it has been used to clean wounds on the battlefield.

Volume and frequency   Most people have very little idea of how much urine they are passing, although they can usually make a guess at how many times they pass it. We've already noted that in health, the minimum volume of urine an adult can pass and remain healthy is about 500–600 ml/day (a pint or a little more—see previous chapter) and the maximum on an average fluid intake in temperate climates is about 2–2.5 litres a day (4–5 pints). Of course, if you're in the habit of visiting the pub and like beer rather than whisky, the sky's the limit. Most people pass less urine when they have been sweating a lot, especially in hot and above all humid climates, and fluid intake needs to be adjusted accordingly if you take exercise. You'll notice that tennis players at Wimbledon never pass the bottles of lemon barley water (Coke seems to have taken over recently) without drinking, but I've never seen one take time out to pass urine.

However, most normal individuals pass urine four to eight times a day, occasionally at night. The ability to hold urine for 12–24 hours may be useful but (except when very dehydrated) is probably abnormal. In children, ability to hold urine for these very long periods is one of the signs (the children themselves rarely complain of it) of a large, slack bladder whose nerve supply may be disordered.

Unless it is merely a habit or the result of taking fluids just before going to bed, *passing urine regularly at night*, perhaps more than once, is a valuable sign that something may be wrong. It indicates one of two things. Either in older men, the prostate gland at the base of the bladder is enlarged, which results in a need to pass urine more frequently and at night as well as some difficulty in starting and stopping the stream. Or, that the usual fall in urine volume during the night is not taking place, and that probably the volume of urine to be passed has increased, that is, the concentrating power of the kidney has become impaired.

The commonest cause of loss of concentrating power is kidney failure, in which the volume of urine usually goes *up* rather than down, as one would expect. The reasons for this are complicated and I won't go into them here. More rarely the rest of the kidney is working normally, and thus kidney failure is not present; but the inner part of the kidney, the medulla, where the concentrating mechanism is found, is affected in isolation. Even more rarely, there can be a deficiency of the hormone ADH (antidiuretic hormone), or exceptionally, resistance of an otherwise normal kidney to the action of ADH. This may run in rare families of 'water drinkers'; only males are affected.

Passing urine very frequently, especially if accompanied by pain in the urethra and bladder and a feeling that the bladder has not been emptied, is the classical symptom of *urinary tract infection*. This is a very common complaint, especially in women, and is rarely associated with kidney failure in adults. In older men, frequency may be the main result of partial obstruction of the urinary outflow from the bladder by an enlarged prostate, but will usually be accompanied by a poor stream, an inability to start or stop passing urine as promptly as before, and perhaps dribbling between times. Although kidney failure can result from prolonged obstruction from a large prostate, there is often little in the way of symptoms in someone whose kidneys are already badly damaged by this.

Incontinence of urine, in an adult individual previously continent, is obviously abnormal. In old people it may be the only sign of a urinary tract infection, and will disappear if this is treated. Apart from prostatic problems in older men, women may become intermittently incontinent with problems of prolapse of the uterus, which pulls down the bladder and urethra with it. Dementia may, of course, come to light as incontinence, but this will not be the only complaint. None of these is associated with kidney failure.

In *children*, the problem is much more complicated. Girls usually become 'dry' at night about the age of two and a half, boys by four or four and a half.

Many normal children have 'accidents' at school, or if unable to find a toilet. Most children who are late in gaining control over their bladders, or particularly those who develop enuresis (wetting at night) having once been dry, have problems which relate to family conflicts, to moving house or school, or other anxieties. However, these children need to be checked to make sure the enuresis is not the result of a urinary tract infection, and if the infection persists or returns may need to be looked at further. A very small number may already have kidney damage.

Boys may be born with a narrowing in the urethra which conducts urine to the outside from the bladder (see Chapter 4) and observant mothers—especially those who have had boys before—may notice that their stream of urine is poor or dribbly.

Appearance of the urine

Surprisingly little information can be gained from looking at the urine. The colour depends very much upon the volume, concentrated urine being darker ('stronger') than the dilute urine passed if a good deal is drunk.

Bleeding from the kidney or the urinary tract of course requires investigation. The appearance of fresh blood, or dark-brown altered blood, indicates a problem. *Old blood* in the urine is often likened to tea in Britain and to Coca Cola in North America, and may be difficult to distinguish, especially in retrospect, from normal concentrated urine. The appearance of fresh blood is always alarming to the individual concerned.

There are very many causes of blood in the urine (haematuria), many of them benign, but the commonest cause of fresh bright red blood in the urine is a severe urinary tract infection, which is temporary and not serious. Some medical treatments, particularly warfarin or other anticoagulant drugs, may be a cause. Fresh blood in the urine is often the result of problems in the bladder and ureters, or even the urethra, and will require investigation by looking into the bladder (see below). Bleeding from further up usually produces brownish urine, including from the kidney itself.

Occasional drugs and foods will turn the urine a strange colour. The best known of these is purple urine from eating beetroot ('beeturia'). Some proprietary medicines contain methylene blue, which turns the urine a greenish colour. In jaundice the urine will often be dark, or even yellow from the pigment retained because the liver is obstructed or unable to get rid of this substance.

Odour

Normally, fresh urine has very little *smell*, but on standing the urea in it breaks down to ammonia, which gives the characteristic odour most people associate with it. If infected, urine may smell foul even when first passed, and this is a valuable sign for the doctor (see Chapter 3). Some foods (for example, asparagus) or drugs (for example, penicillins) give unusual odours to the urine.

Frothy urine

Normal urine froths a little, but persistent frothing which will not flush away is abnormal. This may indicate that there is an excess protein (albumin) in the urine, which when beaten up by the passage of the urine stream, forms a stable foam—just as egg white will when beaten. Frothy urine may also be seen in jaundice because of the bile salts in the urine.

Swelling of the body (Plate 1)

This used to be called dropsy, but this name has all but died out. The term usually applied in medicine is *oedema* (which is simply Greek for swelling). Swelling is an important sign of some kidney diseases, especially those affecting the glomerular filter. Sometimes the name of the *nephrotic syndrome* is given to the coincidence of swelling, a lot of protein in the urine, and low protein in the blood (see below).

The first and earliest sign of swelling from kidney disease is puffiness around the eyes in the morning. Often this is worse in one eye, that which has been underneath whilst sleeping on one side. This gives the clue to the fact that this swelling will slip down to reappear as puffy ankles by nightfall. If severe, then the whole face will be swollen, the abdomen distended by fluid, and the ankles and even the thighs swollen whatever the time of day. The arms may show the 'Popeye' sign, especially if in bed for a period, i.e. the swelling collects round the elbows and forearms to give the appearance of Popeye's arms. This is made more obvious if the swelling is the result of protein loss in the urine, because the upper arms often lose muscle and become thinner. In bed the ankles will become less swollen, but the bottom and back will become waterlogged (or more accurately, salt-and-water-logged).

Of course, there are many other commoner causes for swelling, especially of the ankles, besides kidney disease. The commonest cause of swollen ankles is varicose veins, or after a clot has formed in the veins of the calf ('phlebitis').

Heart failure, liver disease, and gastrointestinal troubles may all cause generalized swelling, and one of the most powerful ways of distinguishing one from the other (apart from the doctor examining you, of course) is to test the urine for protein (see below).

Pain

Pain, as usual, is a signal that all is not well. However, many serious conditions are quite painless, in kidney diseases as in other branches of medicine.

The commonest pain related to kidney disease is *pain on passing urine*. This may be confined to the act, continue between attempts to pass urine, or be associated with pain just above the pubic bone, over the bladder. It may also be associated with pain higher up, at the waist or behind, over the kidneys. This usually indicates, if the problem is an infection, that the infection also involves the kidneys; the reverse is not true: i.e. the absence of pain in the kidney does not indicate that the infection is confined to the bladder.

The next best known form of renal pain is *renal colic*. This is a misnomer, since this pain actually comes from the *ureter*, not the kidney. It begins in the side, or upper abdomen, and appears to travel down into the lower abdomen, becoming nearer the midline. It may radiate into the pubic region, into the penis or testicle in men. The pain comes and goes, and is very severe; many people who have had several painful episodes testify that their 'renal' colic was the worst. Usually this pain is associated with something jammed in, or passing down the ureter: commonly a stone, often very tiny.

True *kidney (renal) pain* is much more difficult to localize, but pain from the kidney itself is usually felt in the back and side, about the level of the waist-band. This may be difficult to distinguish from the much commoner pains arising from structures in the spine, or elsewhere in the back. Many patients have taken their pain from the orthopaedic clinic to the kidney clinic, or vice versa! Occasionally, one finds pain which becomes worse on taking large volumes of fluid, especially with alcohol. This may indicate that there is an obstruction to the urine flow which becomes important when the volume of urine is greater.

Non-specific symptoms

Many of the symptoms of kidney disease, and particularly kidney failure, are called *non-specific*. That is, they are common complaints which would not of themselves make you or your doctor think of kidney trouble or kidney failure. As someone's kidneys fail, they become gradually more anaemic, mainly because the output of EPO from the kidney falls (see Chapter 1). At first they will not look pale, but will notice increased tiredness, and a falling off in physical performance, about which they may or may not be tempted to complain, especially if they are overworking and expect to be tired.

Apart from the underlying pallor, patients with kidney failure may notice that they are becoming browner than before and that they tan more deeply and remain tanned longer than previously. Their skin may also become drier, and they may notice one of the most distressing symptoms of renal failure, itching.

The bone problems of kidney failure may result in general 'aches and pains' especially upon walking, sometimes more specifically located in the bone. Cramps, especially at night, may be a problem, and larger coarse jerking movements of the limbs ('restless legs') a real problem. The symptoms of chronic kidney failure are dealt with in more detail in Chapter 3.

Investigation of the kidneys

One can learn relatively little about the kidneys or their function by direct examination of your body unless kidney function is very impaired. Enlarged kidneys can, of course, be felt, but this is relatively uncommon. Swelling (oedema, dropsy) is easily detectable (Plate 1) but the kidney performance is not so accessible as, for example, the heart. Doctors rely, therefore, a great deal on the results of tests. Indeed modern nephrology is at least in part the creation of the various diagnostic tests which are now available, most of which have been introduced within the past twenty years.

Simple blood and urine tests

The first level of tests are those performed upon *blood or urine.*

'Stick' tests on the urine   *Urine* has been studied as a sign of general disease since the days of ancient Greece, and no physician up until 250 years or so ago would have been seen without his urine bottle. However, this type of study was really divination by urine examination to determine the future, on the same level as examining the entrails of birds. Only in the past 200 years or so has it been studied to give specific and useful information about the kidneys.

The simplest urine tests are the familiar 'stick' urine tests for blood or protein on a casual specimen of urine (Plate 2), in which paper strips are dipped into the urine and the colour read off from a chart on the bottle. In some circumstances, particularly diseases of the glomerular filter such as glomerulonephritis or a nephrotic syndrome (Chapter 5) patients, or parents, will need to make regular tests of their own urine using the strips.

These strips are extremely simple to use. The strip is dipped in the urine and the colour of each of the small squares of paper containing the chemical reagents is read off against a chart. This way the presence of protein, blood, glucose, or bile can be detected, and the acidity of the urine measured. In the case of protein, the square is yellow if no albumin is present, and turns a deeper and deeper green if it is present in greater quantities than normal. This colour is compared with five squares on the bottle which show the colour expected for 0, $+$, $++$, $+++$, and $++++$ on the test. These colours and scores can be approximately related to different concentrations of albumin in the urine; it is best to test the urine at the same time each day, to eliminate variation dependent upon the volume of the urine: the first sample in the morning is usually the most concentrated and is convenient.

The original test for protein, however, was the tendency of urine with albumin in it to coagulate when heated, just as an egg white does when boiled. The test with the sticks (e.g. Albustix (R)) are sometimes still confirmed by boiling acidified urine, to check that it shows a visible coagulation, but usually a specimen will be sent to the lab for more precise measurement, if the stick test is positive.

Absence of blood or protein (albumin) in the urine can be reassuring, but their presence only opens the gate wide, and suggests further investigation (Chapters 3 and 4).

Urine cultures   When a urine infection is suspected, a culture of the urine to see if dividing bacteria are present, and a look at the urine down a microscope are needed. To culture germs from the urine, the test must be done immediately, and the urine collected with some precautions to avoid contamination, which in essence means wiping or washing the outside of the urethra before passing urine, and avoiding contamination from the foreskin in men or the vulva in women. The urine is then collected by putting the jar into the urine stream when you have already begun to pass urine, and then taking it out of the stream again. This is why this type of urine specimen is often called a 'mid-stream' specimen; it requires a little skill to get this right!

Twenty-four hour urine collections   More elaborate urine tests (for example, to examine the total amount of albumin that is being lost in the urine) usually require a full 24-hour urine collection, that is all the urine you pass in a full day and night, but not more. This is a nuisance to collect and may be difficult or embarrassing at work. The best way to conceal a 24-hour urine bottle is in an ordinary shopping bag. The problem is to carry it will you *everywhere*, so that no urine is lost. It will also help the doctors if you tell them if some *has* been lost—it will help them interpret the result. An effective manoeuvre for men is to put a safety-pin through the top of the fly so one is reminded about the fact that a 24-hour collection is in progress. Twenty-four-hour urines are usually required for estimation of protein loss, or creatinine clearance, or for assessing the amount of calcium or sodium in the urine.

Blood tests   Kidney doctors are generous with blood—your blood—and the amount taken may seem alarming unless one remembers that you have 6 litres (12 pints) in all. The tests are directed at many general and specific objectives; the general aim is to estimate the level of various substances concerned directly with kidney function. The most important in relation to the kidney's excretory function are the waste products *urea* and *creatinine*. Both are nitrogen-containing compounds which the body has to get rid of through the kidneys. Neither are important in themselves as poisonous substances, but act as useful markers of kidney function, as they are relatively easy to measure and the concentration in the blood rises as the kidney's function is compromised (Figure 8).

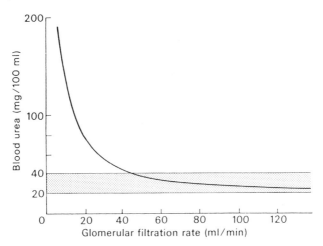

Figure 8   The rise in the concentration of urea in the blood with a fall-off in kidney function. Note that about half the kidney function needs to be destroyed before the concentration rises above normal, but that after this it rises rapidly. The creatinine in the plasma behaves in the same way, and is often used as an index of kidney function: the upper limit of normal is 110–120 μmol/l, and rises to about 1000 μmol in severe kidney failure.

For example, a creatinine concentration in normal plasma is more or less 100 units (in fact, micromoles per litre). In end-stage kidney failure the level is about 1000 or more. Thus following the plasma creatinine concentration is a useful way of judging kidney function. When this value is near normal, however, it is not very good at predicting kidney function, but becomes more accurate as the level rises (Figure 8, and see next paragraph). Other measurements will be made, usually lumped under the heading of 'electrolytes', which relate to the kidney's regulatory capacity, e.g. salt (sodium), bicarbonate, potassium, or chloride.

Tests of specific kidney function may be carried out which require the patient's co-operation. The commonest is a measurement of the amount of water being filtered at the glomeruli—the glomerular filtration rate, or GFR. This is estimated in one of two ways.

First, a 24-hour urine can be collected, with a blood sample at some point during the collection. Creatinine is normally excreted by filtering alone, without too much interference from the tubules. The rate at which it is eliminated from the body, corrected by the concentration in the blood (the 'clearance' value), gives a good approximation of the amount of water being filtered by the kidney, called GFR; it is as good (or bad) as the accuracy of the 24-hour urine you supply.

The other way the GFR can be measured is to give the kidneys a load to get rid of and measure how fast they do this. The usual method is to inject a minute quantity of an inert radioactive compound which can be measured easily in the blood at various times as it disappears; this has the advantage that no urine is required, but the disadvantage is that the test takes several hours of your time, and requires an injection and several blood samples—usually three or four samples will be taken.

A test less frequently done is to see how concentrated a urine the kidney can form. This involves thirsting overnight, then during the morning of the next day until 5 per cent of the body weight has been lost (as water): the urine is collected at this time. The test only works if you don't cheat by having some water during the thirsting period.

What do your kidneys look like?

As well as wanting to know how well your kidneys work, your doctors will want to know what they look like, or even how many there are, or where they are. Some people have only one kidney, in some each kidney is divided into two almost separate kidneys, and kidneys can be found down in the pelvis as well as in the usual places.

Ultrasound scans Frequently the first test done is an *ultrasound* scan of the kidneys (Plate 3). This will be familiar to many women from examinations taken of the baby during pregnancy, and involves no injections or radioactivity, and is perfectly safe. Jelly is spread on the skin and the ultrasound probe moved over the skin over the abdomen and side; the kidneys can be seen on the screen, and pictures of the screen taken as needed by the person doing the ultrasound. This test is very quick, and is especially good at picking up obstruction of the kidney. It tells the doctor immediately if a kidney is missing, misplaced, shrunken, or enlarged. New techniques for assessing the bloodflow in the arteries to and from the kidney by ultrasound are now available, and likely to be increasingly used in the future.

X-rays of the kidneys X-rays of the kidneys are still a commonly used investigation. The most usual of these was the *intravenous urogram*, or IVU (Plate 4), although this is used less and less nowadays as ultrasound and CAT scanning (see below) have improved. This involves some preliminary precautions to ensure that the bowel is empty of gas (which may obscure the pictures), and (for patients with normal or nearly normal kidney function) a low fluid intake to ensure concentrated urine. It is important however, if your kidney function is impaired, that you do *not* thirst or have a purgative, because you will become dehydrated since your kidneys will not respond appropriately. The contrast medium, which is translucent to the eye in the syringe, but is opaque to X-rays and will show up on the X-ray plates, is usually injected into a vein in the arm. Especially with big doses, an unpleasant sensation of flushing may be experienced, and the contrast may be painful if the injection is difficult and it goes outside the vein. Pictures are taken shortly after the injection, and up to two hours later; and one after the bladder has been emptied. If obstruction of the kidneys is suspected then later pictures may be needed. A moving X-ray machine may be used to show the kidneys more clearly ('tomography').

A more trying X-ray is that of the bladder, the *micturating cystogram*, or MCU (Plate 5). This is most often needed in children and adolescents, but occasionally may be needed in adults. It is designed to see the flow of urine out of the bladder, and whether any urine refluxes back up to the kidneys. A fine catheter is passed, with sterile precautions, into the bladder, and the radio-opaque contrast medium is run in. The catheter is then removed, and the patient asked to pass urine, whilst still or cine pictures of the bladder and urethra are taken. Many patients find this whole procedure trying and embarrassing, and find it difficult to pass their urine when requested. However, at the moment the information can be obtained in no other way. Sometimes *pressure measurements* will be taken at the same time from bladder and rectum, using very fine probes.

In special instances, X-ray pictures of the blood vessels to the kidney are required. This is a *renal arteriogram* or angiogram (Plate 6). This requires the patient to lie quietly, and drugs are given as a premedication so that the patient is sleepy, or even asleep, during the procedure. Under an injection of local anaesthetic, fine tubes are passed into the large blood vessels in the groin, and manipulated up to the kidney inside the blood vessel. Radio-opaque contrast is then injected into the kidney. Again, a flushing feeling may be experienced following the injection. After the procedure, firm pressure is kept on the blood vessels and the patient needs to remain lying down to allow the minute punctures in the blood vessels to heal. Usually it is possible to go home at the end of the day, unless bruising or bleeding are a problem.

Other X-ray techniques include the *CAT scan* (computerized axial tomography) (Plate 7). In this, an X-ray source rotates slowly round the area to be examined and a computer constructs a picture of the whole of the 'slice' of the body that has been scanned. Usually, no radio-opaque contrast need be injected, but this may be given to improve the quality of the pictures and to aid their interpretation. This gives excellent pictures of soft tissues which are impossible to see on ordinary X-rays, including the kidneys. For a CAT scan you need to be within the machine while it goes round, and some people find this rather claustrophobic.

MRI scans   A newer imaging technique is the *MRI (magnetic resonance imaging) scan* (Plate 8). This involves no injections and no exposure to X-rays, relying on signals put out by the atoms in the body after they have been exposed to a sudden strong magnetic field, which is quite harmless and undetectable. Because the atoms in different cells and tissues are arranged differently, the signals can be interpreted by computer into pictures of the organs within the body. The test again involves being within a machine and lying still, which some people find trying, and at the moment most machines are very noisy. Both MRI and CAT scanning show soft tissues which do not show up on conventional X-rays, and MRI of the kidney shows the internal anatomy of the organ rather well.

Isotope scans   Use is also made of *isotope scans* of the kidneys. In these a minute amount of radioactive material (it carries no danger) is injected to show up the blood as it passes into the kidney and passes through into the urine. Other substances are taken up by the kidney and can be used to show a static picture of the organ (Plate 9). This is particularly good at showing up tiny scars in the kidney. It must be emphasized that even though the compound is taken up by the kidney and stays there some time, the radioactivity decays and becomes negligible within hours or days.

Pictures for this type of scan are taken with what is called a gamma camera, which is a large array of detectors which put the picture together. This is very large and heavy and some people are afraid it will fall on them, or feel unhappy whilst lying under it. Much of the size of the apparatus is in fact lead shielding so that the pictures will not be blurred by outside radiation.

Kidney biopsy

This important test is often done in the investigation of diseases affecting the glomerular filter. It involves taking a very small piece of kidney out using a needle so that it can be examined in the laboratory, and the pattern of damage (if any) of the glomerular filter determined.

What does it involve?

Usually the biopsy will be done in the morning, so that you can go home in the evening after the test is completed. Blood checks will be done beforehand to ensure that your blood clots normally, and an ultrasound will be done to check the position of your kidneys. It's wise to have no more than an early cup of tea, and to skip breakfast, in case you feel sick later, which happens occasionally.

Usually, you will be given a premedication half an hour to an hour before the biopsy is planned, with a drug designed to relieve anxiety which will also make you sleepy; some people even sleep through the test itself. You will need to lie on your stomach with your head and abdomen supported by pillows. The kidneys are located using an ultrasound machine (see above) and their position marked. Local anaesthetic is injected at the point selected, which is on the back about four inches from the midline, between your ribs and your pelvis, to numb up the tissues; normally the left kidney will be biopsied.

A thin exploring needle will next be inserted to check the exact depth of the kidney, and when the doctor is satisfied that the kidney is located, the biopsy needle is put down the same track and a small core of kidney tissue removed (Plate 10). Often two cores will be needed, sometimes only one.

After the biopsy you will need to lie quietly for some hours to ensure that there is no bleeding from the kidney, and for the effects of the premedication to wear off; someone will need to be available to take you home. During the afternoon you should drink and the first urine you pass will be examined—often it contains a little blood, but this is not a cause for concern. If your urine becomes bright red and remains so, you may have to stay in overnight. Very rarely, enough blood is lost that a transfusion may be required, and obviously you would need to stay in overnight for this.

The result of the biopsy is usually available within a day or two.

Summary

In the kidney clinic, or kidney ward, it is common to spend more time having the investigations than seeing the doctor! But he or she needs this information as well as what you tell him or her to best understand what your kidneys look like and how they are performing, and thus what is going on.

3 Potentially treatable causes of chronic kidney failure: how can we prevent kidney failure?

An ounce of prevention is worth a pound of cure

Anon.

How many people get kidney failure?

Kidney failure is not nearly so common as a cause of death or medical problems as (for instance) heart and blood vessel disease, or cancers as a whole, which each cause more than 200 000 deaths a year each in the UK alone. In the UK, about 7000 people reach end-stage kidney failure each year. This figure may not seem large for the whole country, but kidney failure is more common than a number of diseases which are well known to the public—for example muscular dystrophy and multiple sclerosis.

Many people dying of kidney failure are over the age of 70 or 80 years, and a notable feature of kidney failure is that the *incidence* (the number of people getting the problem for the first time) rises steeply all the way from 15 to 90 years of age. This means that at any one time the *prevalence* (that is the number of people around in the population with a particular problem) is about 40–50 000 in the UK who have conditions which will lead on to kidney failure. Again a large proportion—perhaps half—will be over the age of 70.

What causes kidney failure?

There are several common and almost another 100 rare diseases which may lead to progressive destruction of the kidneys. The main ones are listed in Table 1. In this chapter, I will first discuss those for which there are treatments which will either cure or cut down the numbers of people developing kidney failure.

An important point is that the predominant causes of kidney failure vary with age. It is not surprising that in childhood, inherited disorders and those

Table 1   Causes of kidney failure

Specific treatment not available yet	*Specific treatment or prevention effective in at least some cases*
Glomerulonephritis	Glomerulonephritis
IgA nephropathy Mesangiocapillary gn (MCGN)	Membranous nephropathy Focal segmental sclerosis (FGS) Goodpasture's disease (anti-GBM) Lupus nephritis Vasculitis
Inherited disorders	Inherited disorders
Polycystic kidneys (PKD) Alport's syndrome Childhood (recessive) PKD	Oxalosis Cystinosis
Amyloidosis Sickle cell disease Renal cancers Haemolytic-uraemic syndrome Small kidneys of unknown origin	High blood pressure Vascular disease of the kidney Obstruction of the urinary tract Kidney stones Reflux nephropathy Diabetes Analgesic abuse

present from birth (congenital disorders) should be the commonest, whilst in the elderly, blood vessel diseases and obstruction due (for example) to enlargement of the prostate should be most usually found. Another important point is that in a number of people, which increases with age, kidney failure is found at an advanced stage with very small or scarred kidneys, and the cause of the kidney failure is never determined.

In some respects, which particular disease happens to cause kidney failure does not matter very much, since all forms of kidney failure have much in common. However, it *does* matter whether there are treatments which will arrest the progression of the disease, and also when in some diseases, the kidney is only one of several organs affected. For example, in the case of diabetes, systemic lupus erythematosus (SLE), and vasculitis in adults, for all of which there are treatments which will reduce the impact of the kidney disease, and some rare conditions in children such as oxalosis (hyperoxaluria), what happens in the rest of the body may be at least as important or even more important than the kidney itself, especially if there is little that can be done to deal with the other problems. In some conditions, such as inherited disorders, there may be implications for the family as well as for the patient.

There are a number of conditions for which at least some effective treatment is available. This does not mean that *nobody* with these conditions goes into kidney failure—many do; but it is possible to postpone kidney failure indefinitely in at least some.

We must admit, however, that the opportunities for preventing renal failure remain unsatisfactory at the moment. It would be good if early detection of kidney diseases could lead to effective treatment, and in some cases (for example obstruction of the urinary tract) this is in fact so. However, screening (for example) for protein in the urine is not much use, since small amounts of protein in the urine are common in childhood and in young adults, and usually of little long-term significance in most people.

Kidney failure from forms of glomerulonephritis

We can do little to slow down or prevent kidney failure in people with a number of chronic forms of glomerulonephritis (see Chapter 4), although this is an area under intense investigation at the moment. Given that this is the single biggest cause of renal failure in young adults, we shall not make big inroads into the number of individuals going into kidney failure until this problem of progressive glomerulonephritis is solved. However there are a number of other areas in which prevention is possible and effective.

A benign form of nephritis: steroid-response nephrotic syndrome ('minimal change' disease)

First, because it presents in a very similar way to many other forms of glomerulonephritis which may progress, it is worth mentioning a condition which, although it can cause a lot of worry and have many complications and is susceptible to treatment, does *not* lead to kidney failure. Although it is commonest in childhood it may occur at any age up to 80 years or beyond.

In this condition, which presents with the swelling characteristic of the nephrotic syndrome (Plate 1), one sees in a kidney biopsy that the glomerular filters appear normal or nearly normal under the ordinary light microscope, although the more powerful electron microscope may show subtle changes at higher magnification. Because of this the condition is usually given the name of 'minimal changes'. The reason for the leakiness of the glomerular filters to protein and the appearance of a nephrotic syndrome is not known, and blood is almost always absent from the urine. It responds well to treatment with a variety of medicines, including corticosteroids like prednisolone, and also drugs used to suppress immune responses such as cyclophosphamide (Endoxan) and cyclosporine (Sandimmun). However it tends to relapse and although these relapses usually become less and less frequent with time, in a few people they may persist for decades and it may be necessary to take treatment long-term, and not just with each attack. The responsiveness of the condition to steroid drugs leads to it being called 'steroid-responsive nephrotic syndrome' especially in younger children in whom it is not thought necessary to do a kidney biopsy. It is also called 'nephrosis' although this term is going out of use.

Membranous nephropathy

In this form of glomerulonephritis, some of those affected heal spontaneously whilst others progress, without treatment, into kidney failure. Although we know associated factors which go along with progression of the disease, in any individual it is impossible to say whether this will happen or not. This makes selecting patients for treatment difficult, but a good proportion of those with progressive disease appear to respond to treatment with drugs such as prednisolone, cyclophosphamide (Endoxan), or chlorambucil (Leukeran). The treatment usually lasts several months but the ideal protocol to get the best results without the side-effects of the drugs has yet to be worked out.

Focal segmental glomerulosclerosis (FGS)

This can look very like the 'minimal change' disease discussed two paragraphs ago, with a relapsing nephrotic syndrome responsive to treatment, and indeed about a quarter of children and a fifth of adults who show FGS in their kidney biopsies behave much as though they had 'minimal change' disease, suggesting that the two are to some extent related. However, if untreated, about half of children and two thirds of adults with the appearance of FGS in their kidney biopsies go on to develop kidney failure, usually within 5–10 years. Some of these patients can be helped either by prednisolone, cyclophosphamide (Endoxan) or cyclosporine (Sandimmun). Cyclophosphamide is usually only given for up to three months to avoid side-effects, but cyclosporine may be given for many months or even years.

Kidney failure associated with high blood pressure

Most people are aware that high blood pressure (hypertension) is associated with a higher than normal risk of blood vessel problems both in the brain and in the heart, and that this is one of the commonest causes of disease and death in 'developed' societies. However the kidney has a role as both a generator of high blood pressure, and as a victim of damage when high blood pressure is present.

What will I notice if I have high blood pressure?

There are few symptoms which can be identified as being specifically due to hypertension. Headache, particularly a persistent headache, present on waking in the morning, may be a feature. Some people develop, or suffer, more severe migraine when their blood pressure rises. If heart disease is present at the same time, then heart failure may be noticed early, with breathlessness, inability to lie flat because of shortness of breath. However, the great majority of people with a blood pressure high enough to cause problems over months or years will notice nothing unusual; and this is why it is important to measure the blood pressure from time to time even in people who are apparently well, or in those who are complaining about something entirely unrelated.

What determines blood pressure?

'Blood pressure' usually means the pressure within the *arteries*, i.e. arterial blood pressure. This pressure is the product of three factors (Figure 9):

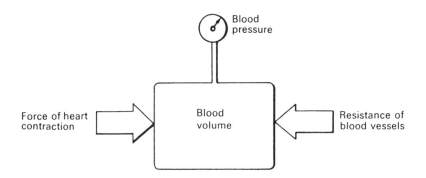

Figure 9 The three components of the blood pressure (see text).

(1) the energy of contraction of the heart pushing the blood out into the circulation. This can vary with both rate and force of contraction of the heart;

(2) the resistance of the small blood vessels in the periphery, which is largely a function of the diameter of these vessels. They can dilate or constrict in response to hormones or nervous signals and vary their resistance;

(3) the volume of blood in the circulation. This is normally constant, but obviously falls if bleeding (haemorrhage) occurs, or if salt and water are lost in excess. Equally, the circulation can be over-filled if salt and water are retained in excess, or rapid blood transfusion is given.

How do we measure blood pressure?

As more and more people with high blood pressure, and with kidney diseases, now measure their own blood pressure, we will go into this in a little detail.

Two blood pressures are usually measured; the *systolic* and the *diastolic*. By convention the systolic is written first, and the diastolic second, thus 130/80—in some countries this is written 13/8. The units are millimetres of mercury (mmHg) from the height of the column of mercury in the measuring apparatus. For those more used to car tyre pressures, 100 mmHg equals about 2 pounds per square inch (p.s.i.).

The *systolic* pressure corresponds to the peak pressure during the active phase of ejection of blood from the left ventricle of the heart, the *diastolic* to the trough of pressure between phases of ejection. The *mean* blood pressure is obviously somewhere between the two (Figure 10). To measure the pressure accurately one needs to put a needle into the artery and read it directly on a

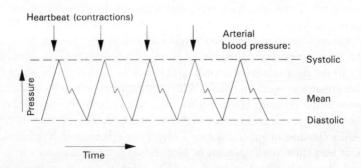

Figure 10 The variation in arterial blood pressure throughout the course of one heartbeat. The systolic (higher) and diastolic (lower) blood pressures are shown.

pressure transducer. This is actually done in some situations, for example during and immediately after heart operations.

For routine day-to-day use however, the familiar blood pressure cuff is used (Plate 11) which gives a fairly accurate reading, usually by following the sequence of noises heard over the artery with a stethoscope, whilst the artery is compressed or decompressed with the inflatable cuff upstream from the point of listening. Most often, blood pressure is measured in the arm, near the brachial artery which can be found and listened to just above the elbow. The point where a noise is first heard for each beat of the heart, when the pressure in the cuff is lowered, approximates to the *systolic* pressure; and the point where this sound suddenly goes soft, after gradually increasing in amplitude, approximates to the diastolic.

Many people (even doctors!) find the sounds not too easy to interpret, and today, a number of relatively cheap machines are available, which after putting on the cuff and inflating, do the work for you by sensing the vibrations in the blood vessel (oscillometry), with a direct display of the numbers. These are much easier to use, and now that they give more accurate readings than in the past, are in wider use (Plate 11).

One important point is that the size of your arm will influence the levels obtained if a standard cuff 13 cm (4½ inches) wide is used; the fatter the arm, the greater the over-reading.

The normal blood pressure

What is 'normal' blood pressure? A moment's thought about the factors which determine blood pressure will indicate that blood pressure will not be constant, but will vary all the time. Pressure readings taken continuously by devices worn all the day, have given startling data which indicates just how much the 'normal' blood pressure can vary from deep sleep on the one hand to violent exercise or excitement on the other. A completely 'normal' individual might have temporary variations as large as from 110/60 to as high as 220/140 during a relatively normal day.

This presents us with a problem. What is usually meant by a 'normal' blood pressure is the pressure taken, usually in a sitting position, during the day whilst you are at rest and neither frightened nor excited. Such conditions are not easily obtained in either a doctor's surgery or especially in hospital! Even then, at least three readings must be obtained on different occasions to give a general idea of the blood pressure, and the value of a single examination— unless it is extreme—is quite small. Usually the blood pressure obtained at the first visit to the doctor, and especially after being admitted to, or attending

36 *Potentially treatable causes of chronic kidney failure*

hospital will be 10–20 mmHg higher than the figures obtained on subsequent visits.

The vicious circle of high blood pressure and kidney damage

Usually high blood pressure has no obvious cause, and is called 'essential' hypertension. In this situation, you will often have a history of high blood pressure in your family, and this commonest type of blood pressure is probably a result mainly of an inherited susceptiblity. However this can also be provoked or made worse by lifestyle or diet, particularly the intake of salt (which tends to raise blood pressure), potassium and calcium (which tend to lower it) and maybe stress. Alcohol also raises the blood pressure in the long term.

However, in addition high blood pressure may be the result and the outward sign of other diseases, and the commonest situation in which high blood pressure is found as a result of identifiable disease elsewhere is in *diseases of the kidney*. The importance of this observation lies in the fact that high blood pressure in turn damages the kidney (Figure 11). Thus, a vicious circle can be

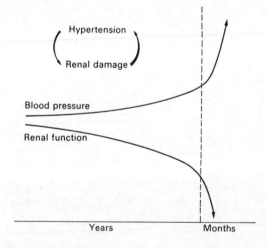

Figure 11 The vicious circle of high blood pressure and kidney damage. However you enter the circle, whether from having high blood pressure first, or by developing a kidney disease which gives rise to high blood pressure, the end result is the same: progressive kidney damage and a steadily rising blood pressure. At some point, which varies in time and at different levels of blood pressure, the whole process accelerates and a rapid rise in blood pressure occurs with damage to blood vessels throughout the body, particularly in the eye and in the brain.

set up, either from essential hypertension, but more commonly from renal disease leading to secondary high blood pressure. Only if this vicious circle is broken by treatment can kidney function be preserved. The final stages can be very rapid and even if the patient does not succumb to a stroke, kidney function can decline to nothing within a very few weeks. This phase of hypertension, whether primary (essential), or secondary to kidney disease, is often referred to as 'malignant' hypertension, although the term 'accelerated' hypertension is preferable. It is characterized by severe damage in the small blood vessels all over the body (including the kidney), which can best be seen in the back of the eye through an ophthalmoscope; by the appearance of proteinuria, if not already present, as an indication of the renal damage; and finally, if untreated, by convulsions and eventually death.

The treatment of high blood pressure

The treatment of high blood pressure, both as a complication of kidney disease and as a cause of kidney failure, is the most important aspect of the prevention of kidney failure at the moment. In many countries, including the UK, screening for blood pressure is given high priority by governments and by doctors.

We already know that the death rate from the most severe forms of high blood pressure (accelerated or 'malignant' hypertension) has decreased to less than one-quarter of what it was in 1960 and is still falling. We know also that treatment of less severe but still serious hypertension cuts the number of strokes and heart attacks suffered by hypertensive individuals. Evidence is now accumulating that treatment of severe blood pressure also cuts the amount of renal failure. We do not yet know if treating relatively mild but significantly high blood pressure—which is much more common—will improve the figures still further.

Another important point is that high blood pressure is common in people with kidney failure from other causes, and it is almost certain that control of this type of high blood pressure at least slows the progression of renal failure, even though the underlying condition is still progressing.

What does treatment of high blood pressure involve?

There are a number of things that you as a patient can do to help lower your blood pressure. In some people these avoid the need for blood pressure lowering medicines altogether, although this is unusual if your blood pressure arises from kidney trouble.

Diet and high blood pressure   Obviously the most important factor in the control of high blood pressure is *salt*. Moderate reduction of salt intake is often successful, either alone or in combination with a diuretic or drugs to reduce the blood pressure (see below). All hypertensives should watch their salt intake and, if they are overweight, try to bring their weight back to normal. As well as an effect in the actual reading dependent upon the size of the arm, there is a real reduction in blood pressure with weight loss, and of course your heart has to work less hard in daily activities if you are not carrying the equivalent of a sack of potatoes around with you all the time.

Lifestyle and high blood pressure   There is no doubt that a pressurized life-style leads to sustained rises in blood pressure, but whether these become permanent has been much debated. Conversely, one can 'train' oneself to reduce blood pressure by a variety of techniques, from simple measures to deep meditation. Any person with high blood pressure who continues to smoke is genuinely inviting suicide, and despite the difficulty of overcoming this socially sanctioned addiction the goal must be achieved. Nicotine patches will help to break the addiction to playing with the cigarettes themselves, and a gradual reduction in the use of the patches will wean you off addiction to the nicotine. Finally, although a modest alcohol intake is possibly even beneficial, excessive alcohol definitely raises the blood pressure. Each week, no more than about 25 units (each unit is 8–10 ml of alcohol, i.e. half a pint of beer, a glass of wine, or single 'short') should be taken, and for women only 14–20 units/week.

Treatment of high blood pressure with medicines   For most patients with both primary and kidney-induced hypertension, treatment centres round the use of diet and medicines to lower and control the blood pressure. From what we know about the mechanisms of blood pressure (Figure 9) three approaches are available to achieve this:

(1) reduce the force with which blood is put out from the heart;

(2) lower the resistance of the small blood vessels in the periphery;

(3) reduce the volume of blood in the circulation.

All three can be used, and in practice two or three are often used together, so that smaller doses of the individual drugs may be used to achieve the desired reduction in blood pressure, and thus minimize the side-effects. Although this means you may have to take several pills instead of one, this is very important. This is because the biggest problem in the treatment of blood pressure is not to control blood pressure, but ensuring that if you have high blood pressure you keep on taking the drugs, most of which have side-effects which are much more common at high doses. Details of the medicines most commonly used and how they act are given in Box 1.

Conclusions

The treatment of high blood pressure has been one of the success stories of medical treatment in the last 30 years, only second in saving life to the antibiotic revolution. The main problem has been to seek methods of treatment which do not have unacceptable side-effects. Now that there are available agents which satisfy this need and are also effective in lowering the blood pressure, it might be thought that the problem has been solved. Not so. Surveys in the UK show that at least half those who *could* benefit from treatment of their severe high blood pressure still do not receive adequate treatment, even ignoring the possibility that milder levels of blood pressure might benefit from treatment. Studies in the USA show better control and fewer complications of high blood pressure in patients followed-up in special clinics, compared with those treated by physicians in practice.

Why do we sometimes fail? First, about one-third of people with treatable severe high blood pressure are still unidentified, since those suffering from it have never had their blood pressures taken. The complicated issues of the human and cash value of screening versus its cash cost cannot be debated here, but the medical necessity for seeking out undiagnosed severe high blood pressure are quite clear. More worrying is the fact that only about half the *known* hypertensive patients have their blood pressure controlled adequately. There are several reasons for this failure, but the crucial one seems to be inadequate supervision of the treatment, and inadequate explanation of the role you, the patient yourself, must play in maintaining a normal pressure, and the fact that blood pressure treatment is usually a contract for life. This remains a challenge which must be accepted—and dealt with—immediately.

Major blood vessel disease affecting the kidneys

Only recently have we realized just how common narrowing of the major blood vessels supplying the kidneys (renal artery stenosis) may be as a cause of kidney failure (Plate 12). Part of this is attributable to the increased numbers of people surviving into old age, and the increasing numbers of the elderly being investigated and treated for kidney failure.

Box 1   Medicines used to treat high blood pressure

Drugs acting on the cardiac output

The principal drugs in this category are a group called beta-blockers. This refers to their action in blocking a particular set of nerve endings which (amongst other actions) stimulate the cardiac output and heart rate. Thus, a reduced workload for the heart is induced, often with a slow pulse which does not rise with emotion or exercise. Drugs in this category usually have names ending in -ol, such as oxprenolol (Trasicor), atenolol (Tenormin), metroprol (Betoloc), and so on. The dose is usually quite low to begin with, but depending upon the severity of the hypertension and the response, the dose may be increased steadily. Side-effects differ, but some may give rise to tiredness, wheezing, nightmares, impotence, and cold fingers. As a result, these drugs, although effective in small doses, are usually not used alone or in severe hypertension.

Drugs acting on the resistance of the small blood vessels

Drugs, called *ACE inhibitors*, which block the production of the constrictor hormone angiotensin (see above and Chapter 1) are of particular value in high blood pressure complicating renal disease, in which renin and angiotensin levels are usually high. These drugs usually have names ending in -pril, such as Captopril (Capoten), enalapril (Innovace), lisinopril (Zestril, Carace), and so on. These and other similar drugs are now very widely used in the treatment of kidney-induced high blood pressure, especially as they reduce the amount of protein in the urine, which may be a risk factor for further renal damage, and the way they act seems particularly favourable to benefiting damaged kidneys (see diabetes below). They have few side-effects except that in some people a persistent dry cough is induced which makes it impossible to continue the drug.

A third 'family' of medicines used for high blood pressure are a group called *calcium channel antagonists*, which directly act on the muscle in the blood vessel wall. Their names often end in -ine such as nifedipine (Adalat) and amlodipine (Istin). Although very effective and widely used, these have one bad side-effect in that they cause severe flushing and headaches in many people. This however can largely be eliminated by using slow release (SR) preparations, which also have a longer lasting effect, and which most people can tolerate without problems. Some people also get troublesome ankle swelling when taking these drugs especially amlodipine, and a very few get swelling of the gums.

A final 'family' of medicines used in the treatment of blood pressure are the *alpha-blockers*, which block the nerves which make the muscle in the small vessels contract. These drugs usually have names which end in -azosin, such as prazosin (Hypovase) and doxasosin (Cardura) which has a longer action. They have few side-effects but may interfere with potency in men.

Drugs acting to reduce the blood volume The principal drugs here are the diuretics. Given the central role that salt plays in high blood pressure, it is not surprising that drugs which lead to increased sodium and chloride excretion are effective in treating blood pressure. In addition, some diuretics, such as the thiazides (e.g. Navidrex), also have a direct effect in dilating the small blood vessels and thus are useful in two ways in treating hypertension. These have few side-effects but can deplete the body of the valuable potassium, and may also cause impotence in men. More powerful diuretics such as frusemide (Lasix) are usually needed when patients with impairment of renal function develop high blood pressure, and in advanced kidney failure very big doses may be needed to achieve an effect. Diuretics are rarely effective on their own in patients with renal disease and blood pressure, because they push the renin levels in the blood— already high—even higher as they deplete the volume of circulating plasma by increasing salt and water excretion. Hence, other drugs are necessary in combination to lower blood pressure.

Drug combinations in blood pressure treatment

This re-introduces a crucial point. Usually, it is better to attack high blood pressure by one, two, or three of the approaches just outlined. Although it may mean that you have a row of pills to take, rather than just one, the great advantages of avoiding the side-effects outweigh any problems of remembering to take them. Only in mild blood pressure, a thiazide diuretic, which is also a dilator, will be used alone. For somewhat more severe blood pressure this will be combined with another drug such as a beta-blocker. In more severe hypertension, a beta-blocker will be combined with a dilator such as captopril, nifedipine, or prazosin, with or without a more powerful diuretic such as frusemide. This triple combination attacks blood pressure from all three points of origin, and may allow smooth control of even severe blood pressure as a complication of advanced kidney disease.

Kidney failure usually results as only one manifestation of blood vessel disease which is usually present throughout the whole arterial system, not just the kidneys, which is strongly associated with prolonged smoking, and with a family history of blood vessel disease. There are no specific symptoms or signs of kidney failure from blood vessel disease, but today, all patients with some degree of kidney function impairment and blood vessel disease elsewhere—for example in the heart, legs or brain—are considered as possibly having narrowing of the arteries to the kidneys if they have any degree of kidney failure. The diagnosis is made by doing an arteriogram (see Chapter 2), less commonly by doing an MRI (Chapter 2) angiogram, which has the advantage of not requiring an injection into the artery. Other clues that renal blood vessel disease may be present are unequal-sized kidneys without another explanation—for example reflux (see below). Usually, patients with kidney failure from this cause have high blood pressure, but this is not always the case.

The importance of finding narrowing in a major vessel to a kidney, especially if it is effectively the only kidney still working, or the one which is doing most of the work, is that it is usually progressive. Fortunately, quite often this can be reversed or arrested by one of several procedures.

The first of these is dilating the blood vessel using an inflatable balloon passed on the end of a catheter in through a major artery elsewhere; this is called *balloon angioplasty*, and is the preferred treatment in the often elderly patients with kidney failure from widespread blood vessel disease, including the main artery to the kidney.

The second approach is to do a *surgical operation* called *autotransplantation*. In this operation, the kidney is taken from its natural site. The artery is operated on whilst the kidney is flushed and cooled as in a standard transplant operation (see Chapter 8) and after the narrow portion has been enlarged or removed altogether, the kidney is transplanted to the large blood vessels in the pelvis as in a standard transplant. The ureter is not touched, however.

Alternatively, a *bypass operation* can be done, but this is rarely applied in older patients because of the poor quality of the blood vessels. It is more often used in younger patients whose problem from the narrowed artery is high blood pressure, without kidney failure. Using either a tube of artificial material such as either Dacron (R) or Gore-Tex (R), or a piece of the patient's own vein (usually from the leg) a new channel is sewn across the blockage in the artery to the kidney or provide a bypass round the obstruction. A variation is to split the narrowed vessel, and widen it by sewing in a 'gusset' of vein or artificial material. If artificial material is used then the patient may need to take anticoagulant drugs such as warfarin, or antiplatelet drugs such as aspirin afterwards, to prevent clotting of blood on the material introduced into contact with the circulating blood.

Urinary tract infections, reflux and chronic pyelonephritis

Urine infections are very common, especially in women, and only *very* rarely indeed are an indicator of a condition which will lead on to kidney failure. In many women the symptoms (of pain and frequency of passing urine with burning) are confined to the bladder area ('cystitis') although in some attacks there is tenderness and pain also over the kidneys, and in a few shivering shakes (rigors) which indicate that the germs have escaped from the urine and the kidneys into the blood stream. Nevertheless, this is overwhelmingly a benign condition, although cystitis may be a tremendous nuisance in women who suffer frequent attacks.

However, in a minority of children and young women, recurrent infections are a sign that the urinary tract is not normal. The problem is to try and detect the members of this tiny minority amongst the very large numbers of people who have infections.

Which patients with infections get kidney failure?
Reflux nephropathy and 'chronic pyelonephritis'

In a small minority of children and young people with recurrent infections is a condition called *reflux*, or more accurately, *vesico-ureteric reflux*; this is the commonest single cause of kidney failure in children and adolescents. These problems start very early in life, in most cases probably before birth, and the damage is done by the end of the first year of life in most cases.

Reflux is associated with abnormalities of the kidney which are present at birth, called renal *dysplasia*, i.e. abnormal growth of the kidney. The most likely picture of what happens is that, even before birth, as a result of a defect in the valve at the junction of the ureter and the bladder, urine can pass backwards up to and into the kidney as well as out through the urethra when the bladder contracts (Figure 12): hence, vesico-ureteric reflux, or reflux for short. At this time and in infancy, the kidney is poorly protected against the entry of urine into its substance back along the tubes of the nephrons, and urine can begin scarring if it breaks out into the substance of the kidney, as it will if pressure within the bladder and ureters is high. This is particularly likely if, in addition, there is obstruction, which can occur in the urethra in boys (Plate 5) and at the bladder neck in girls (see next section).

As with various forms of glomerulonephritis, one puzzle is to understand why only some patients with reflux but without obstruction nevertheless go on to develop progressive scarring of the kidney and kidney failure, whilst others do not. Those who do, usually develop both high blood pressure and quantities of protein in their urine, both of which are therefore valuable clues as to the likely outcome. Some people, despite grossly scarred kidneys, maintain their kidney function over many years, although they may be prone to some other problems—for example, if they are women, developing high blood pressure when they take contraceptive pills, or during pregnancy.

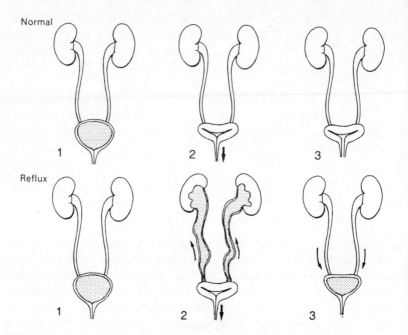

Figure 12 Reflex of urine during the passage of urine. At the top, events in a normal individual are shown. The valve between the bladder and the ureter does not leak (1), and the bladder empties completely (2). After passing urine (3) the bladder is empty.

In contrast at the bottom of the figure the situation in reflux is shown. During the passage of urine, this refluxes back up to the kidney (2) either on one side only or on both sides, as shown in the diagram. After passing urine, the bladder relaxes and the urine in the ureters falls back into the bladder which is thus never emptied and provides an easy reservoir for infection should any germs gain access to the urinary tract from below or from the bloodstream.

Actual reflux of urine itself tends to go away during childhood as the bladder wall gets thicker with time, but of course the scarring of the kidney persists, even if it is not progressive. This type of coarsely scarred kidney used to be called 'chronic pyelonephritis'. It is important to identify those children with reflux even without obstruction, because they need treatment with long-term antibiotics to prevent the infections, which are often without any symptoms, and which may help to damage the kidneys. In a few children with persistent infections despite this treatment, it may be worthwhile re-plumbing the incompetent ureters back into the bladder by an operation, although it is not clear whether this achieves anything more than cutting down on the frequency of infections.

Obstruction of the urinary tract

Obstruction, especially if accompanied by infection (which is frequent) leads to destruction of the kidney behind the obstruction, and if present on both sides renal failure will eventually appear. Obstruction of the urinary tract can occur at almost all levels in the urinary tract (Figure 13), and from a variety of

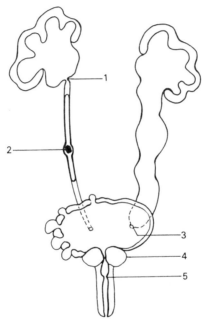

Figure 13 Possible sites of obstruction in the urinary tract. (1) is at the junction of the pelvis and ureter, often called a PUJ (pelvic–ureteric junction) obstruction. This is usually congenital, but may only come to notice later. The pelvis will blow up and the kidney substance thin. (2) is obstruction in the ureter. This is usually acquired from a variety of causes within the ureter (stones), in the wall (tumours, inflammation) or pressing on the ureter (tumours, inflammation. (3) shows an obstruction at the junction of the ureter and bladder. This is often congenital, but may be the result of surgery to cure reflux, if the ureter is sewn in too tightly. It may also result from a thick bladder wall, as shown on the left of the diagram, resulting from obstruction at sites (4) and (5) in the outlet from the bladder and the urethra. (4) is usually the result of prostatic enlargement in males, and (5) either congenital anomaly (urethral 'valves') or as the result of infection, often from repeated gonorrhoea. If the obstruction at these sites persists, then the bladder wall thickens with small sacs bulging out at weak places in the wall, as shown on the left of the bladder in the diagram.

causes: at the bladder neck and urethra, especially from prostatic enlargement in older men, and from congenital abnormalities in young children, especially boys, as just discussed in the last section; at the junction of the ureters and the bladder, usually as a result of thickening of the bladder wall, or again from congenital abnormalities; in the ureters from a variety of causes, especially stones forming within them or from pressure from outside by growths; or at the junction of the ureter and pelvis from congenital narrowing or stones.

The detection and treatment of urinary tract obstruction is one of the goals of the investigation of a patient suffering from chronic kidney failure (see below). If found, relief of obstruction can convert the situation from one of advancing, progressive renal failure into stable renal insufficiency compatible with a good future and normal life. Clearly, the earlier the obstruction is detected the better: hence the need to investigate patients with persistent or current infections for abnormalities of their urinary tract, especially young children. Operations to cure reflux or treat infection associated with it also may prevent renal failure.

Acquired obstructions

Kidney stones do not usually cause kidney failure, often because they come to notice early on, by reason of the pain they cause. The usual stones are made of calcium oxalate or calcium phosphate, or combinations of the two. In some people there is an excess of either calcium or oxalate in the urine, and this can be treated by increasing fluid intake and thus urine output, modifying diet, and by medicines such as diuretics to reduce calcium output—but in hyperoxaluria (see above) stones form repeatedly, as well as calcium oxalate deposits in the kidney which destroy its substance. Another rare inherited cause of kidney stones—fortunately much less serious and a very rarely causing kidney failure —is *cystinuria*—not to be confused with *cystinosis* discussed later. Cystin*uria* is a recessively inherited condition (see Box 2), by which cystine is not re-absorbed in the kidney tubules as it should be as it is concentrated up as the urine is formed; since it is not very soluble, crystals and then stones form. It can usually be treated successfully by increasing urine volume and making the urine alkaline with bicarbonate, or by making the cystine more soluble using the drug penicillamine.

Some very large stones however (often called 'staghorn' calculi from their shape), may be associated with infection and slowly destroy the kidney without any pain. These stones form in infected urines, and the infections are almost impossible to get rid of in the presence of the stones.

There have been many advances in the treatment of stones during the past twenty years. Stones can be broken up using the machine known as the litho-tripter, in which the patient lies whilst shock waves are focused on, and passed through the stone, which fragments. The fragments are then passed over the next few days, sometimes with a little blood, sometimes not. Occasionally a further treatment will be necessary to break up the biggest fragments. Another technique, sometimes used before lithotripsy, is to drain a kidney obstructed by a stone through a tube inserted into the side via a needle and wire, and then left in place. An instrument can then be passed down the same track from the side, and the stone broken up by direct application of the shock waves. It is rare today to have a full operation to remove a small or medium-sized stone, although the very big 'staghorn' stones may have to be removed this way.

Prostatic enlargement affects 30–50% of men over the age of 60 and is increasingly common above this age. The signs of this may creep up so slowly that despite really quite gross changes in ability to pass or control urine the sufferer often does not complain to his doctor. Commonly it is difficult to begin passing urine, the stream is poor and slow, and at the end dribbling occurs. There is often a need to pass urine quite frequently, both during the day and at night. In the great majority of affected men, there is no obstruction affecting the kidneys and kidney failure is not a problem. Turned the other way round however, prostatic obstruction is one of the commoner causes of kidney failure in old age in men. Increasing attention is being paid to screening for problems in men at risk.

Fortunately, a number of treatments are available for benign prostatic en-largement. It is often very difficult to decide when or whether to treat, depend-ing on the severity of symptoms and the amount of disturbance they are causing. This is an individual matter: some men find getting up at night a couple or more times a major burden, whilst others treat it as a minor incon-venience. Also, any treatment seems to be associated with a considerable response rate, probably because the evolution of the problem is so slow and erratic. Medicines, in particular drugs called alpha-blockers which are used in bigger doses to treat high blood pressure (prazosin (Hypovase (R)), doxazosin (Cardura (R)) can diminish symptoms and postpone or avoid the need for specific treatments. However, the 'gold standard' specific treatment remains the Trans-Urethral Resection of the prostate, or TURP, and in individuals who already have problems with kidney function as a result of their prostatic problem, this is almost always necessary. In this procedure, under a general anaesthetic a scope is passed up the urethra and using a blade through the same instrument, the enlarged prostatic tissue around the urethra is chipped away. This completely removes the obstruction, but often does not affect the frequency, if this is a problem. Disadvantages of this operation are a very small chance of incontinence afterwards, and effects in sexual function. Because after this procedure, retrograde ejaculation into the bladder occurs, the subject is sterilized. Also, there is about a 10% incidence of impotence after it.

A number of other new treatments are under trial at the moment. The two most discussed are the use of a new drug finasteride (Proscar), which stops the production of the derivative of the male hormone, testosterone, which promotes the prostatic enlargement. This is achieved without any effect on testosterone itself, so that potency and sexual characteristics are not affected. The second approach is to heat the prostate, using microwaves or other techniques. A third approach is to dilate up the narrowed urethra with a balloon, with or without putting in stent to maintain the increased channel. Trials have shown all three treatments to result in an improvement in symptoms, and in the case of the first two a reduction in prostate size, but the longer term effects of both procedures are still being examined.

A minority of enlarged prostates with obstruction are shown to be the result of *carcinoma of the prostate*, which is now the second commonest cancer of men after lung cancer. Clues to the presence of a growth in the prostate in someone with prostatic symptoms are a raised level of a test in the blood for *prostate specific antigens (PSA)*, and a suspicious pattern on ultrasound of the prostate. A biopsy of the prostate can be done to determine what the pattern is down the microscope. Fortunately, a number of treatments are available for this common cancer, although results are still not nearly as good as one would like.

Retroperitoneal fibrosis (RPF) is a rare type of inflammation which occurs near and around the ureters, typically in middle aged males. It is not clear what triggers the inflammation, but it may relate to weaknesses in the major artery arising from the heart, the aorta, and the condition may be improved by treating with steroids such as prednisolone, with or without operating to move the ureters forward out of the way of the obstructing inflammatory tissue.

Other infiltrations which can involve the ureters behind the peritoneum as they run down to the bladder include spread from various tumours, and the outlook and treatment obviously depends upon from where the mass of cells has come.

Inherited obstructions

This may affect the upper part of the urinary tract in children and young adults, and if diagnosed early and treated by operation or by blowing up a balloon to dilate the narrowing, renal function can be preserved. The commonest place to find such a narrowing is at the junction of the pelvis of the kidney with the ureter (see Figure 13). This can be present on one side only, or on both sides which is of course more serious since both kidneys are put at risk. If the narrowing is important but not critical, it may be many years before it comes to light. In some children, the obstruction is so severe that the hugely swollen pelvis and kidney can be felt in the abdomen, or even seen!

Often, if inherited obstruction affects the lower urinary tract, reflux of urine back into the kidney occurs at high pressure into the kidney, with the effects discussed above (see pyelonephritis, kidney scarring, and reflux). The commonest form of inherited obstruction is in boys in the early part of the tube from the bladder to the end of the penis—the urethra. These urethral 'valves' as they are sometimes called (Plate 5) are relatively easy to treat once their presence has been recognized; however in the meantime damage to the kidney can occur. One important sign in baby boys with this type of obstruction is that their stream of urine is poor and hesitant compared with normal boy babies, and mothers may notice this. They may also suffer frequent kidney and urine infections because of the obstructed urine pooling in the dilated bladder, ureters, and kidneys.

Pain killers toxic to the kidney (analgesic nephropathy)

The third area for prevention is the abuse of analgesics (pain-killers). A group of patients who have taken very large amounts of mixed analgesic pills or powders for many years may go into renal failure from damage by the drugs to their kidneys: *analgesic nephropathy*. These pills contain aspirin, phenacetin or its relatives, and codeine or caffeine.

The kidney damage usually takes the form of an inflammation of the tubules and surrounding tissue of the kidney, with eventually complete destruction and separation of the tips of the medulla of the kidney, so-called 'papillary necrosis'.

Most of the individuals with analgesic nephropathy take large amounts of mixed analgesic pills which they get over the counter in the chemists for reasons other than their pain-killing effects—particularly in the belief that they will be calmer, have more 'pep', or sleep better with the pills than without. These individuals are commonly middle-aged women, but men may also be affected. A high intake for many years is needed to produce damage, with 10–20 pills per day; ordinary use of analgesics does not lead to renal damage, but anyone taking self-prescribed analgesics every day should be seeing someone about the habit, or the reasons for needing the analgesics. If the analgesics are stopped the patient frequently becomes dependent upon drugs such as benzodiazepines (e.g. Valium) which are (relatively) innocuous, or alcohol, which is not. However, a number of unfortunate individuals have analgesic damage to their kidneys because of a necessary high intake of analgesics—for example for severe arthritis.

It now seems clear that the drug phenacetin is the culprit, and this has been banned in most countries, so that prevention of this variety of kidney failure is now well on the way to being completed in most countries. However it is still common as a cause of kidney failure in (for example) Belgium and Australia. The evidence is good that stopping the analgesics leads to an arrest in the fall-off in kidney function and then some return. Conversely, restarting the pills, or continuing with them leads to more kidney damage.

Diabetes

Diabetes is a disease which can affect almost every part of the body, including the kidney. Usually, the kidney, eye, and nerve complications do not appear until 10 years have passed from diagnosis, and peak at about 19-20 years from onset. Diabetes is one of the commonest causes of kidney failure, especially as more older diabetics are surviving longer, and developing kidney problems.

We now know that very good control of the blood sugar in diabetics slows or stops the appearance of both the eye and the kidney complications of diabetes. This may explain the good news that both these complications have been becoming less and less frequent in the past 20-30 years in young diabetics who need insulin. Now, we can make deliberate attempts to limit the damage, but this involves a lot for the diabetic, with three or four injections of insulin a day, and extremely careful control of the blood sugar on the glucose meter, to make sure it does not fall to low and a 'hypo' results.

We also know today that, even after kidney damage has appeared in someone with diabetes—for example they already have protein in their urine—treatment with ACE inhibitors (see Box 1, treatment of high blood pressure) will slow the decline in their kidney function, and at least postpone entry into kidney failure. This may be because of the way these drugs, as opposed to other drugs which lower the blood pressure, act on the pressures within the glomerular filter itself.

One problem which still remains is that these manoeuvres do not prevent some of the other problems of diabetes—for example the blood vessel disease which may affect the legs and the heart.

Systemic lupus erythematosus

This is a disease which results, as with glomerulonephritis, from abnormalities in the immune system which protects us against invasion by foreign organisms. It affects predominantly young women and adolescent girls. Unlike primary glomerulonephritis, almost every organ in the body can be affected, but particularly the kidney, the brain, the joints, the skin, and the membranes around the heart and lungs. Often other organs are affected, particularly the joints and skin, for months or years before the kidney is damaged, but sometimes the kidney is affected from the beginning. The glomerular filter may show anything from the mildest damage to the most severe forms of nephritis, and the disease can change during its course from one to the other. The kidney disease generally comes to attention because of proteinuria, frequently enough to cause swelling and a nephrotic syndrome (see above).

The disease responds well to steroid drugs such as prednisolone, often combined with azathioprine (Imuran) or cyclophosphamide (Endoxan). Problems in the long term mainly relate to side-effects of these drugs (see Chapter 8 for discussion), since relapses may be seen years—or even decades—later if the drugs are stopped or reduced. In a few fortunate patients the disease appears to 'burn out', and all treatment can be stopped. In a minority of patients renal failure appears, and surprisingly, often the disease activity decreases at this point. However some patients with lupus need treatment with prednisolone and other drugs throughout and after dialysis treatment.

Vasculitis (polyarteritis, polyangiitis)

This name implies inflammation of blood vessels, and this is what the condition arises from. Yet again, the problem is a malfunction of the immune system, so that blood vessels of various sizes are inflamed, break down, and become clotted, with obvious implications from the tissues depending on them for their supply. When small vessels are those affected, then the kidney is a major target for damage. Patients with vasculitis are generally ill, with weight loss and fever, and frequently have a spotty rash since the skin is often affected. Joint trouble may also be present with pains and swelling in the joints. The lungs are often affected, and in some forms of vasculitis (often called Wegener's after the doctor who described them) the sinuses, the ears and the nose may be affected. So far as the kidney is concerned, in contrast to lupus, in general the kidney does not leak large amounts of protein in this condition. Thus a nephrotic syndrome is not seen, although blood is always present in the urine. Renal failure is often severe, right from the outset, and dialysis may be needed straight away.

As with lupus, the disease is quite responsive to treatment to suppress immune responses with prednisolone and cyclophosphamide, and kidney function can be recovered in most cases. Thus the long term problem, again as with lupus, is often one of side-effects from the drugs needed to keep the disease suppressed.

Most forms of vasculitis are commonest in older patients, above the age of 50, but one particular form of vasculitis which is almost confined to children, is called *Henoch-Schonlein purpura*. Purpura describes the spots which characterize the affected skin, and as well as the common joint problems, pain in the abdomen from problems in the bowel occur. Strangely, this form of the disease usually does not respond to prednisolone, but fortunately it is usually a much milder disease in the kidney than other forms of vasculitis in older patients. Nevertheless, some children and adolescents do have severe nephritis and despite treatment go into kidney failure.

Cystinosis

Cystinosis is an inherited disease characterized by a defect in the transport of an amino acid (which therefore forms a normal part of proteins) called cystine, out of cells. Thus *all* tissues can be affected although the kidney is the main organ affected during childhood. However, if the renal failure is successfully treated, for example by a kidney transplant, then other organs may be affected: the eyes, the liver, diabetes may develop, or the brain may be affected.

Inheritance

Cystinosis is inherited as a recessive condition (see Box 2 in Chapter 4) i.e. as a result of having both a father and a mother who are carriers for the disease. Thus the chances of further children being affected are 1:4; of being themselves carriers, 2:2.

Treatment, if started early, can prevent kidney failure and the other problems that cystinosis brings. This consists of a substance called phosphocysteamine, which allows the cystine to escape from the cells. The progress of the condition and its treatment are followed by looking at the amount of cystine in the white cells in the blood. Obviously this strategy requires early identification of children with the disease, which is often difficult.

4 What causes kidney failure? Causes as yet without a specific treatment

Hardness of the kidneys . . . is either not well cured,
or cured by no means

Giuglielmo Saliceti (1211-1277): *Durities in Renibus*

Progressive forms of kidney disease for which specific treatments are not yet available

Glomerulonephritis

Fortunately, we already know from Chapter 3 that not all forms of glomerulo-nephritis lead to kidney failure, and that of those types that do, not everyone affected takes this course. However, in all groups of young adults with kidney failure who have been studied, the commonest single cause of kidney destruction are one or another of the group of conditions known collectively as *glomerulonephritis.* This is not true of children, or of the elderly, as we have noted above.

What is glomerulonephritis? Glomerulonephritis is the name for inflammation of the kidneys, particularly (but not exclusively) affecting the glomerular filters. An older name is *Bright's disease*. The exact nature of this group of disorders remains unknown, but we do know that in general they arise from problems with the reaction of the body's immune system, which protects us from invasion by bacteria (germs), viruses, fungi, and yeasts which live all around us. In various ways, this defence mechanism comes to attack, not invading organisms, but the body's cells, tissues, and organs themselves. Thus one approach to treatment is to try and inhibit the immune system of the body, and thus moderate the attack. Immediately of course we run into the problem that this will render you more liable to infections, and some other complications which depend upon other functions of the immune system. Fortunately, not all forms of glomerulonephritis go on to destroy the kidney—many can heal completely, perhaps because the immune attack switches off, or even if they return repeatedly, may still leave kidney function intact.

How do you know if you have glomerulonephritis? Glomerulonephritis often comes to notice because of changes in the urine, which may be found in someone who is perfectly well, but has their urine tested because of a health check or an insurance examination. Another way glomerulonephritis comes to attention is through swelling of the body (oedema) (Plate 1). Urine may become brown, or bright red, from blood passed from the inflamed kidneys, or very frothy from large amounts of albumin passed in it (see Chapter 2 for discussion). Both are signs that the filters of the kidney (glomeruli, Chapter 1) are damaged, since normally they do not allow either blood or protein to pass. The swelling is a complicated consequence of the passage of large amounts of protein into the urine for a long period—usually weeks or months rather than days. The combination of swelling, large amounts of albumin in the urine and correspondingly less in the blood plasma is usually called the *nephrotic syndrome* (Plate 1). This may arise from a number of different forms of glomerulonephritis, and also from some other systemic diseases which may affect the glomeruli such as diabetes, infiltration with amyloid, or other immune disorders like lupus (systemic lupus erythematosus, SLE) (see Chapter 3). Why a low level of albumin in the blood and protein coming through the kidney leads to swelling with water and salt is still not clear, although the protein passing through the kidney plays a part.

Usually the onset of the nephrotic syndrome and its swelling is slow, so that only gradually do you come to realize that something is wrong. The swelling is usually most obvious in the face in the morning, with puffy eyes and a bloated face, whereas by the end of the day in an upright position the ankles are the are most swollen. In contrast, some forms of glomerulonephritis may start abruptly, and come on within hours or a day or two at most. This is called *acute* glomerulonephritis, is often accompanied by visible blood in the urine, and although it may be very severe for a short while often heals completely. The forms of glomerulonephritis which show only as gradual swelling, or simply with abnormal urine tests, are more often progressive. Obviously, as with all forms of kidney problem, the degree of kidney function will need to be assessed (see Chapter 2).

Do all forms of nephrotic syndrome lead on to kidney failure? Fortunately, no, but because blood and/or protein in the urine, with or without swelling, arise from a number of different types of damage to the glomerular filters, some of which give kidney failure, some do not, some are treatable and some are not, obviously it is crucial to try and find out what type of injury is going on, what the outlook may be, and whether treatment may alter it for the better.

To achieve this a *kidney biopsy* is almost always necessary (see Chapter 2). The small piece of kidney tissue taken out by the needle is examined carefully in the pathology laboratory after staining with various reagents which help to distinguish the various types of glomerular damage. To begin with, it is worth dealing with one form of problem which, although it may lead to blood and protein in the urine and even severe swelling, and for which there is no specific treatment, does *not* lead to kidney failure. This has become much less common in Europe and North America in the past few decades, but is still common in poorer parts of the world.

Acute glomerulonephritis

For this there is no specific treatment, but it usually heals completely, especially when it clearly follows an infection. These infections may be from ordinary germs, such as the sore throat germ *Streptococcus*, or from viruses. The infections are commonly in the throat or lungs, but may also be on the skin, where the skin is moist and insect bites which become infected are frequent. Thus it is often called *post-infectious acute glomerulonephritis* and although blood and protein may persist without any symptoms for months or even a year or two afterwards, usually heals completely. Despite the fact that recovery usually takes place, during the attack the glomerular filter may be severely inflamed, with red urine accompanied by large amounts of protein and acute swelling, and in a few cases even temporary dialysis may be required.

Which forms of glomerulonephritis may be progressive?

However, for a smaller number of people with acute nephritis as described above, and a large proportion of adults with proteinuria or a nephrotic syndrome, the kidney biopsy when examined by the microscope may show one of several patterns of damage which can lead on to kidney failure. They all share the same characteristic, in that it is only *some* people with the same appearance of damage who go on to develop kidney insufficiency. Why this should be so remains a mystery, although we know some features which are more often associated with progress into kidney failure. These include male sex, increasing age, persistence of a large amount of protein in the urine, with or without swelling, and the presence of raised blood pressure. Some additional clues can be obtained by looking at the kidney biopsy carefully—if scarring is already present, then it is not surprising that the outlook is poorer than when it is absent. Surprisingly, the actual degree of kidney function is not a very good predictor of outcome at the beginning of a nephritis, since many people suffer temporary, reversible drops in kidney function which recover within weeks or months, as in acute nephritis.

These conditions all come to attention either with proteinuria and haematuria, often with high blood pressure (see below) without any symptoms, or with the swelling of the nephrotic syndrome.

These various forms of nephritis which may progress have a variety of names which relate to the appearances seen by various techniques applied to the kidney biopsy specimen. Very important, however, is whether within either of these categories, you have a form which is likely to progress or one which, whilst it may persist for a long time, does not lead to destruction of the kidney. It may be necessary to watch kidney function and measure protein in the urine over a period of many months, or even a year or two, to determine which is the case (see Chapter 2).

Unfortunately, although there are a number which can be treated effectively which we have already dealt with in Chapter 3, for a number of forms of nephritis there are as yet no specific treatments for some. The two principal forms of glomerulonephritis in this category are called *IgA nephropathy*, and *mesangiocapillary glomerulonephritis*, which fortunately is almost always abbreviated as MCGN. In addition, as we noted in Chapter 3, some patients with *focal (segmental) glomerulosclerosis*, abbreviated as FSGS or FGS, progress to kidney impairment.

IgA nephropathy (IgA disease)

In this condition there is usually only a moderate inflammation of the glomerular filters, with the antibody called IgA found in the core of the glomerular filters. Whether the IgA causes the damage is not known. It must be emphasized strongly that many children and young adults with IgA nephropathy and prominent blood in their urine do very well and do *not* go into kidney failure. However some children and a number of young adults, usually men, show only modest amounts of protein in their urine and blood on stick testing, but have in addition high blood pressure and do badly in the long run. Often it takes 10 or 20 years before kidney failure appears in this condition, and unfortunately no treatment available at the moment appears to affect the outlook. Obviously high blood pressure should be treated.

Mesangiocapillary nephritis (MCGN)

Unlike IgA nephropathy, which appears to be more common today than 20 years ago, MCGN seems to have become much less common in developed countries over the same period, although it remains much commoner in developing countries in the tropics. It is commonest in children and young adults, although it can be seen in older people. Often it presents with protein in the urine together with blood which is visible to the eye, or detectable on stick testing; often a full nephrotic syndrome and high blood pressure are present.

There is some suggestion that prednisolone may benefit children with this form of nephritis, but this has not been confirmed. In adults, all forms of treatment tried so far seem to be ineffective.

Focal segmental glomerulosclerosis (FSGS)

This usually comes to attention because of a nephrotic syndrome, and seems to be a more severe variety of the condition called *minimal change nephropathy* which does *not* lead to kidney failure (see Chapter 3). Even FSGS itself is not always progressive and may respond to treatment in up to half of children and one third of adults who have this problem. Nevertheless, in the remainder it may be resistant to treatment and lead to a steady, even rapid decline in kidney function.

Inherited disorders of the kidney which lead to renal failure

A number of inherited disorders of the kidney can lead to kidney failure. Today, gene therapy remains a dream which is only just beginning to become a reality (see Chapter 10). Thus there is at the moment no specific treatment for these conditions, and they run their course uninfluenced by interventions. An immediate additional worry for many patients, once they know they have a serious kidney disease which is inherited, is whether or not their families may be affected also, and in what way.

Polycystic kidneys

Polycystic kidneys (Plate 13) is the most common of the two major inherited causes of kidney failure, and is probably the most common serious inherited disease in the population as a whole.

What are cysts?   Cysts are cavities filled with fluid, usually clear, and lined by cells which give the inside a smooth glistening appearance.

Are all cysts in the kidney bad?   Fortunately, no. *Solitary cysts* of the kidney are common and of no significance; they are often picked up on ultrasound examination of the kidney in healthy people. However in *polycystic kidney disease* (Plate 13) the whole substance of both kidneys is replaced by numerous cysts, the remainder being non-functioning fibrous tissue.

How will I know if I have polycystic kidneys?   They may come to attention in various ways: sometimes someone develops kidney failure and they are found unexpectedly by ultrasound examination (see Chapter 2). The kidneys may become so big that one or both can be felt as a lump in the abdomen, and either you notice it yourself, or it is picked up when having a medical examination for some other reason. The cysts may bleed, and the condition may be found during the investigation of blood in the urine. Infection of polycystic kidneys may be frequent or persistent, and the enlargement and cysts found in investigating this. High blood pressure may be found, and the kidneys in the subsequent investigation of this problem. Finally bleeding into the cysts, or infections may give rise to pain in the side, and the kidneys again found to be abnormal on ultrasound when the pain is being investigated. Finally, some people are aware that the disease runs in their family, and that other family members have had trouble from it.

Unless this is the case, polycystic kidneys usually do not come to attention until middle age (see below), and often it takes five to fifteen years from the time kidney function begins to fall from normal before end-stage kidney failure is present. During this time any of the above symptoms may appear or be present; rarely pain is so severe that puncture of cysts, or even removal of one kidney is necessary, but obviously this is to be avoided if at all possible. High blood pressure is frequently seen, and successful treatment of this is believed to slow the progression of the kidney failure. Cysts may appear also in other sites, principally in the liver, and this may be the major source of problems. Only a very few individuals suffer from severe disease of both liver and kidney, and in the great majority of patients with kidney failure from polycystic kidneys the liver cysts cause no problem at all.

How do polycystic kidneys come about?   Polycystic kidneys are an *inherited* disorder, that is they are the result of a mistake in one part of the huge message of DNA present in every cell which describes how to make a human being (see Box 2). Thus, the mistake can be passed on by those who have the problem to their children through the DNA they give them.

Inheritance   The type of inheritance is such that only *one* unit of DNA from *one* parent is needed to ensure that the abnormality will appear: this type of inheritance is called *dominant inheritance*. Thus, since each piece of DNA

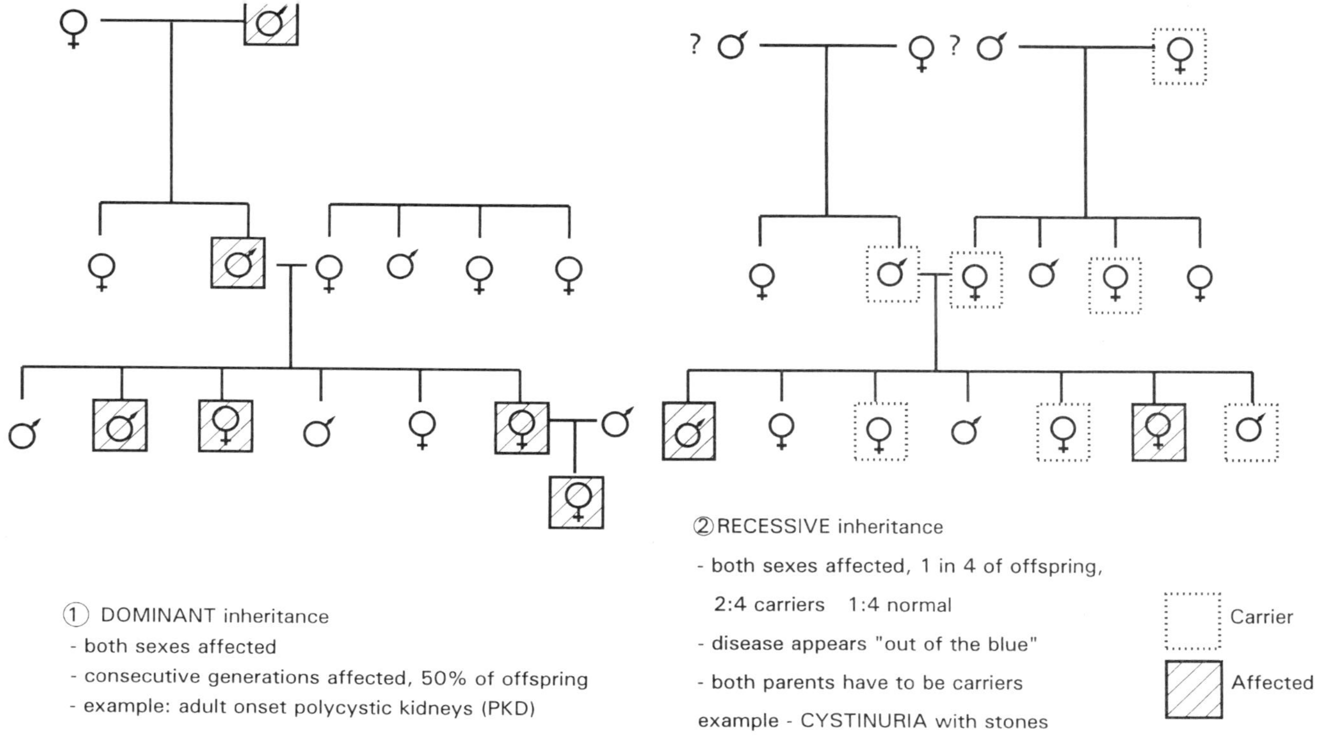
?
?
① DOMINANT inheritance
- both sexes affected
- consecutive generations affected, 50% of offspring
- example: adult onset polycystic kidneys (PKD)
② RECESSIVE inheritance
- both sexes affected, 1 in 4 of offspring,
2:4 carriers 1:4 normal
- disease appears "out of the blue"
- both parents have to be carriers
example - CYSTINURIA with stones
Carrier
Affected

Figure 14 Examples of inheritance of disease. The left panel shows *dominant* inheritance, as is found in adult polycystic kidneys. Only one copy of the gene from one parent needs to be abnormal before the disease will appear. Males are represented by squares, and females by circles (see text). The right panel shows *recessive* inheritance, in which both copies of the gene have to be abnormal before the disease appears.

Box 2   DNA and inheritance of disease

The instructions for 'making' a whole human being are carried by every single cell in the body, including the sex cells, sperm and eggs (ova). These instructions are carried in a message about 3 thousand million units long, formed from DNA, which carries within it the message of at least 100 000 genes which code for different parts and assembly of the body. Genes may be 2000 to 20 000 units long, so the function (if any) of the vast amounts of remaining DNA—sometimes called 'junk DNA' is not known. Each DNA chain is in the form of two chains wound in a double helix, each chain being formed from only 4 different structures called bases, which bind across the helix to a base on the other chain. The corresponding parts thus form a template for the other chain. This DNA is coiled up, the coils coiled again and packed and arranged into 23 chromosomes, each of which is in fact a pair, joined at a waist, with one short arm and one long arm. One of each pair is derived from the mother's egg, and one from the father's sperm, and two copies of every gene are carried. Every time a cell divides, each DNA chain splits and a new chain is created to correspond to the original.

It is obviously possible for errors to creep into this immensely complicated process, which is repeated many times in the growth of the embryo before birth. In addition, if any error affects the DNA in the egg or sperm, it will be passed on to the next generation as part of the instructions. Often the effect of such errors is so large as to be lethal, and a spontaneous early abortion results, but some more minor errors can be passed on from generation to generation. Sperm and ova have only one copy each of the DNA since they are going to form a new individual by fusion together; thus if one bad copy is present in the father or mother, half the eggs or sperm will carry the bad message.

In some conditions, such as polycystic kidneys, even though the affected individual carries only one copy of the defective DNA on one arm of the chromosome, this is sufficient to cause disease. Thus when they form a sperm or ovum with only one arm of each chromosome, half of the sperm and ova will have the defective message and half the proper message. If a sperm or ovum with the bad message fuses with a normal sperm or ovum to form a new individual, if that individual has the bad DNA on only one arm, then disease will appear. This is called a *dominant* form of inheritance.

Alternatively, there are conditions in which *both* the copies on the two arms of the chromosme have to be abnormal before anything happens. In this case, people with only one copy wrong on one arm of a chromosome are carriers, and unless they have children with another carries no disease results. In the case of cystic fibrosis, as many of as 1 in 20 caucasian (white) individuals carries one copy of the erroneous DNA. If a carrier has children by a normal individual, only normal individuals or carriers can result, in equal proportions. However if two carriers mate (in the case of cystic fibrosis a 1:400 chance), the odds are 1:4 that someone with the disease will result because they carry the defective DNA on both copies from father and mother, whilst chances are equally 1:4 that a normal individual with two normal copies of the DNA result. Two in 4 will be, on average, carriers with one abnormal and one normal copy. A most important point is that for any individual pregnancy it will be impossible to predict what will happen—only the chances, on average, can be given. This is called a *recessive* form of inheritance.

These two forms of inheritance apply when the abnormal DNA is carried on one of the 23 ordinary chromosomes. However, men have a XY pair of chromosomes which makes them male whilst women have two Xs: XX. What if the abnormal DNA is on one of the sex chromosomes? There are a few conditions, none of them affecting the kidney, which are carried on the Y chromosome and are inherited only by the sons of affected fathers.

However there is one important disease which can cause kidney failure, *Alport's syndrome* the DNA for which is on the X chromosome. There are also a number of other important inherited disorders carried on the X chromosome, including haemophilia.

If a disease is carried on the X chromosome, things are a bit more complicated. Mothers who are carriers of the abnormality on one of their X chromosomes tend to be normal, or not so badly affected. They can pass one X on to their daughters, but there will be a normal X present and if this is a recessive condition they also will be carriers, but not usually affected. However, 1 in 2 of their sons will receive the affected DNA on what is their only X chromosome—they will get a Y from their father. Thus the sons of carrier mothers develop the full disease. The sons who have the disease cannot pass it on to their sons, because to be sons they must have a Y from their father. However, an affected son can pass on to his daughters his affected X, so that they will be carriers.

There are other, uncommon, modes of inheritance of diseases but these need to be discussed with a doctor who is an expert in the field.

(gene) is carried in duplicate, if you have polycystic kidneys with one normal and one abnormal copy of the gene, for each child you father or bear, there is a 1 in 2 chance they will get the abnormal piece of DNA (gene). Having the gene does not mean inevitably that they will have kidney failure, but eventually about 70–80% do so. One odd thing about polycystic kidneys is that, despite being an inherited disorder, determined at the fertilization of the egg, and present from birth, it usually does not cause any problems until the person with the abnormal gene is 40–60 years of age. However, occasionally it comes to attention in childhood or even infancy, and as just mentioned some fortunate individuals—perhaps 20–30% of those affected—escape major problems until very old age, or escape altogether.

Although we now know the exact sequence and location of the abnormal gene (PKD1) on chromosome 16 (see Box 2) which is responsible for 85% of cases of polycystic disease, what it codes for remains unknown. Another gene, PKD2, is carried in a different part of the DNA (chromosome 4) and finding it is important because families with this type of polycystic disease do not so often go into kidney failure, and when they do, do so more slowly. Until we have both genes fully identified and sequenced, DNA tests are not much better than careful examination by ultrasound of the kidneys in determining whether the condition is present in individuals from many families, although this is likely to change in only a year or two (see Chapter 11).

What does this mean for my family?   Obviously, a question which immediately arises on diagnosis of polycystic kidneys is: what about the rest of the family? Brothers and sisters of the affected individul, if younger, have a 1:2 chance of having it also, since one of the parents will normally have been affected. Older brothers and sisters are less likely to have it, since it is likely it would already be evident in them, but this is obviously not always the case. Each of these adults will need to decide whether they would like to have a screening ultrasound test, and certainly all should have their blood pressures checked—as should everyone in any case in middle age.

By the time the condition is diagnosed, many patients will already have children, as may their brothers and sisters. What should be done about them? This question is a little more complicated, since at the moment until DNA testing is available, it depends to some extent upon *how old these children are.* First, we must remember that apart from treating blood pressure there is no treatment so far which will affect outcome; obviously if one comes to light (see Chapter 11), then the whole position will change. We must ask ourselves whether knowing that a child or young adult has cysts will be better than checking their blood pressure. The knowledge that they indeed do carry the gene for polycystic kidneys can be a considerable disadvantage in applying for jobs and insurance, and no help to them in terms of treatment.

Also, the ultrasound test, whilst very sensitive in picking up cysts of 1 cm (0.4 inches) or so, cannot yet detect those of only a few millimetres (¼ inches). Thus although it is possible to make a strong statement about any individual, whatever their age, that cysts may be *present* in numbers too great for a normal kidney, it isn't possible to say they *don't* have polycystic disease until they are 18-20 years of age. By this time they are capable of making up their own minds about whether they would like to have the test, and that is the advice I usually give to families at the moment.

As far as children of brothers and sisters are concerned, the obvious first thing is to determine whether or not the brother or sister has the condition. If they don't, then the children are safe—the condition cannot 'jump' from person to person. However, if the brother or sister proves to have the cysts without symptoms, then the children may need screening depending upon age, as just outlined for the patient's own family.

Complications Polycystic kidney disease is really polycystic *disease*, since tissues throughout the body are affected. A particular problem is bleeds within the head from small 'blow-outs' on the blood vessels to the brain. These can now be screened for, but this is best done only in families in which someone has already suffered a bleed, or in people who have symptoms suggesting a problem in the cerebral circulation. If easier tests than the current test—an arteriogram by injection into the bloodstream to the head—then it may become worthwhile to screen all patients with polycystic disease, but at the moment the information does not justify the cost and the risk involved. In some other people the valves in the heart may be 'floppy' and leak blood with a heart murmur, as a part of the polycystic disease.

Alport's syndrome

The other main inherited disease causing kidney failure is Alport's syndrome, which is named after the doctor who first described some of the principal features of the condition. It is quite rare, but important as a cause of kidney failure. Alport's syndrome consists of blood in the urine (either on testing or visible), kidney failure, together with deafness and peculiar lenses in the eyes so that eyeglasses are usually necessary. The condition may come to attention with blood in the urine in childhood, followed by deafness by the age of 10, and kidney failure during adolescence or early adult life. Apart from the family history, the appearances of the glomerular filters are characteristic and a renal biopsy in one family member clinches the diagnosis. Unfortunately, there is no treatment that will affect the progression of the disease.

How is it inherited? In over 90% of families, the portion of altered DNA is on the *X chromosome* (see Box 2) of which women have two and men only one; this means that men with the mistake in the DNA are much more severely affected than women, since men have only the one X chromosome, which is abnormal, whilst women have two, only one of which is abnormal (see Box 2). The abnormal DNA codes for a protein important in the structure of the membrane in the filter of the kidney, which accounts for the renal failure;

this protein is present also in the membranes of the lens of the eye, and in the ears, which accounts for the deafness and eye troubles.

Because this is a so-called sex-linked disease, the sons of men affected will be normal, whilst his daughters will all be carriers of the disease. Conversely, the sons of carrier mothers will have a 1:2 chance of being affected with the full disease, 1:2 of being normal. Daughters of carrier mothers have a 1:2 chance of being themselves carriers.

There are other, fortunately benign, inherited conditions which present with blood in the urine but without the deafness and the eye changes of Alport's syndrome. It will almost always be necessary to do a kidney biopsy and DNA testing to see which is present, and naturally all this can cause a great deal of anxiety even if, in the end, the condition turns out not to be Alport's.

A very few families have a different form of Alport's syndrome in which the gene is not on the X chromosome but on an 'ordinary' chromosome. This type is inherited in a *recessive* fashion (see Box 2), so that both parents of an affected person need to be carriers of the altered piece of DNA, and the affected person carries two copies. We are still learning about the evolution and nature of this condition.

Polycystic disease of childhood

An even more rare condition is another disease in which the kidney is affected by cysts, although they look quite different from those of adult (dominant) polycystic disease. Childhood polycystic disease is inherited as a *recessive* condition (see Box 2), that is you need two copies of the mistaken gene before you get any problems; one makes you a carrier. Thus both parents have to be carriers, and any brother or sister of an affected child has a 1:4 chance of having it, and both parents are carriers without symptoms or signs.

Another important difference from adult polycystic disease is that in this childhood form the liver is frequently and severely affected in this childhood form, liver problems may dominate the picture. A transplant of both organs may be needed to deal with this.

Oxalosis

Another rare inherited cause of kidney failure which is almost confined to children is *oxalosis (hyperoxaluria)*. This is a disease which is the result of a deficiency of a protein in the liver which helps break down oxalate, a compound found normally in fruit and tea and coffee, which forms with calcium very insoluble crystals which can damage tissues throughout the body severely.

The age when problems appear is very variable, but most patients with kidney failure already have trouble in childhood. When the disease only makes its appearance in adult life it is usually much more mild and rarely leads to renal failure. The main extra problem is that although the kidney is affected early and severely, because of the high concentration of oxalate in the kidney during the process of forming urine (hence the alternative name of hyperoxaluria), all other organs are at risk, particularly infiltration of blood vessels with the crystals. Thus the only definitive treatment is to transplant a liver as well as a kidney, and this is now the most usual form of treatment for advanced oxalosis. Whether this should also be done early in the course of the disease before real trouble has arisen is a topic which is much debated at the moment.

Inheritance Oxalosis is inherited in a recessive fashion. The most important question that immediately arises is what the chances are of a further child being affected: the answer is (see Box 2) that there is a 1:4 chance of any other individual child having the disease, and 1:2 that they will be a carrier.

Amyloidosis

Amyloid is an infiltration of the blood vessels throughout the body with one of an insoluble group of proteins, called *amyloid*. The body's scavenging mechanisms are unable to get rid of them, so that the insoluble proteins persist and affect organ function, including the kidney which has a large proportion of blood vessels, particularly the glomerular filters. There are two main types of amyloid: amyloid A, also called secondary amyloid, which is a complication of long standing inflammation or infection, such as rheumatoid arthritis, or bone infection (osteomyelitis). The protein, amyloid A is present in the blood in small quantities in health, but the amounts rise enormously during infection or inflammation, this can occur at any age including during childhood. Obviously there is a potential for treatment through treating the disease causing the problem—for example a prolonged infection; however in practice the best that can usually be achieved is to stop further deposition of the abnormal protein into the tissues.

The second type is called amyloid L, also called primary amyloid, and arises from an overactivity of cells in the bone marrow which make antibodies—amyloid L protein is part of the antibody molecule. These abnormalities of the bone marrow cells making antibodies almost always appear over the age of 50.

Treatment is less satisfactory than for secondary amyloid, particularly because this form commonly affects the heart as well, and often the patient with primary amyloid faces major problems with disorders of poor cardiac function and rhythm. However some benefit can be obtained by using medicines which inhibit the abnormal marrow cells—such as prednisolone and cyclophosphamide, or its relative melphalan.

Haemolytic uraemic syndrome

This condition overwhelmingly affects children, although it can affect adults as well. If severe, it leads to a temporary kidney failure which may require dialysis for a few days, or a week or two, but which recovers more or less completely. However in a minority of children and a higher proportion of the small number of adults, kidney failure may be permanent.

The more benign forms follow an attack of diarrhoea related to an infection with a particular bacterium, a form called *E. Coli*, relative of which live in the normal large bowel. The source of the dangerous strain of *E. Coli* is usually contaminated meat, often only partially cooked. Hamburgers have been a source in many patients. In those children and adults who do not recover kidney function, however, diarrhoea is usually absent.

A prominent feature of this condition, apart from the kidney failure (uraemia, see Chapter 5) is a severe anaemia brought about by breakdown of the red cells in the circulation—hence the name of the condition. The kidney failure results from clotting of small blood vessels in the kidney, the result of damage by agents including the bacterium just mentioned, which in turn breaks down the red cells as they pass.

Treatment is dialysis and blood or plasma transfusion; one has to wait and see whether the kidneys will recover or not.

Sickle cell disease

Sickle cell disease is a recessive inherited condition (see Box 2) affecting mainly people of West African origin, although it can be found anywhere from Southern Europe to the Middle East. Thus as a result of the slave trade in the past it is common in American blacks, and West Indian and British Afro-Caribbeans.

The name comes from the appearance of the red blood cells when seen under the microscope, after they have been exposed to low concentration oxygen.

Instead of a smooth round biconcave disk, they form a sickle shape and as a result the blood clots in various small vessels in the body such as in bone, and causes a painful 'sickle crisis' and persistent anaemia because the sickled cells break down more easily. Sickle cell patients are particularly vulnerable to lack of oxygen if they have anaesthetics for operations, or go to high altitudes, or fly in planes. All this results from a small mutation (change) in the gene for haemoglobin which carries oxygen in the blood. Thus the diagnosis of either a carrier or someone affected can be made by looking at the haemoglobin in the laboratory.

Both carriers and people with full sickle cell disease may have problems. In the carriers this usually consists only of pain in the kidney and passage of blood in the urine, occasionally with bits of medulla breaking off into the urine ('papillary necrosis'—see analgesic abuse in Chapter 3), but kidney failure does not appear. The medulla is particularly affected because the oxygen concentration is particularly low there; this is due to the way the blood vessels loop down into it (see Chapter 1). In the disease itself however, kidney scarring results from the repeated episodes when the blood sickles, and in Jamaica as many as one third of sicklers develop kidney failure.

Cancers of the kidney and kidney failure

There are two relatively common tumours of the kidney: Wilms' tumour in children and carcinoma of the kidney in older adults.

Wilms' tumour appears in two thirds of cases before the age of 3 years, and three quarters before the age of 5. It usually comes to attention because of an increase in size of the abdomen which the mother notices, and high blood pressure is common. The condition can be treated by taking the kidney out and by radiotherapy or chemotherapy. Distant spread (metastases) are common but often sensitive to radiotherapy, and results of treatment are very good. However, in a minority of children the condition affects both kidneys, and the child ends up successfully treated but requiring dialysis.

Carcinoma of the kidney is responsible for about 1600 deaths in the UK each year. It is not easily treated, although new agents are being tried at the moment. However in some patients the other (normal) kidney is affected, either with amyloid A (see above) or with forms of glomerulonephritis triggered by the tumour. In these cases, since the other kidney has been removed to eliminate the tumour, renal failure occurs.

Reflux nephropathy and kidney failure

We said in Chapter 3 that reflux of urine and kidney scarring often stops short of kidney failure, or is preventable by operations to eliminate obstruction. Unfortunately in some children and young adults the kidney is very much scarred, tiny, and distorted (Plate 14), perhaps with severe blood pressure, before the condition comes to attention. In this case scarring continues and kidney failure may result. In fact, this type of scarring is the commonest cause of kidney failure in children, at which age kidney failure is of course rare.

5   *What happens to you in kidney failure?*

What happens in kidney failure?

In this chapter we look at what happens to you if you have kidney failure of some degree, which may or may not be progressing, but your own kidneys are still working. Some 40–50 000 people in the UK and maybe as many as 300–400 000 in the USA are in this position. Many will be already under the care of a doctor, but quite a large proportion may not know yet that they have kidney trouble. The majority will eventually require treatment for end-stage disease, by dialysis, by kidney transplantation, or both.

In the previous two chapters we looked at the various diseases which cause kidney failure. In general, at the end it makes little difference which disease you may have, because the same things happen to everyone as kidney failure progresses to some extent, especially when the disease is advanced. However, there are several differences that are important. First, you may have a disease which affects other parts of your body as well as the kidneys, such as diabetes, systemic lupus, or amyloidosis, and problems elsewhere may dominate the scene—for instance, eye difficulties if you are a diabetic, or problems with blood vessels in your legs if you have blood vessel disease. On the other hand, you may have a condition which affects only the kidneys, such as glomerulo-nephritis or reflux. Second, you may have a condition for which treatment is available, and can at least postpone the final destruction of your kidney function. In some people end-stage kidney failure can be postponed almost indefinitely. Third, the availability of treatment, the nature of the disease you have, and how far it has already got will determine how long it takes to get to end-stage kidney failure. In some instances this may be only a few months, in general it will be several years, and in a few conditions it may be as long as 10–20 years or more before real problems arise.

What will I notice if I have kidney failure?

What are your symptoms if you have kidney failure? Although eventually all functions of every cell and tissue of the body are affected in severe kidney failure, the most striking feature of slow destruction of the kidneys is how *little* the patient notices until renal failure is very advanced (unless, of course, the condition itself is painful or leads to symptoms). This is at once a blessing and a curse. A blessing, because people can lead almost normal lives with as little as one-tenth of their renal function surviving. A curse, because the lack of symptoms may result in the individual only seeking help very late in the disease, perhaps in one of the treatable forms of disease which has already gone beyond the point where something can be done to relieve it.

An apparent paradox, which becomes noticeable quite early in loss of renal function is that you may notice you are passing not less urine, but *more*. This extra urine output is distributed throughout the day and night, so that once or even twice you have to get up and pass urine. The reason for this is complex, but a greater proportion of the water filtered by the kidney (see Chapter 1) is excreted as urine, and the ability of the urine to be concentrated at night is limited as part of the general loss in flexibility and ability to vary the composition of the urine in response to demands (Figure 15).

If high blood pressure is present (Chapter 4), it may be symptoms of this which bring the whole problem to notice: breathlessness, morning headache, maybe an ache in the chest on taking exercise. Most patients, however, simply feel 'run down' and tired all the time without being able to be more precise. These vague symptoms are partly the result of the mounting level of toxic substances in the blood—uraemia ('urine in the blood'—see below), and partly as the result of *anaemia*, itself caused because the bone marrow becomes unable to work in the poisoned environment and production of the hormone EPO falls

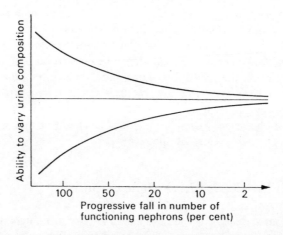

Figure 15 The loss of flexibility of response of the kidney with decreasing kidney function. Eventually the composition of the urine cannot be varied at all, and intake must be kept constant to compensate for this loss.

as the kidneys are progressively damaged (see Chapter 1). Then, as renal failure progresses, the anaemia becomes more profound and paleness becomes noticeable to the patients and to their family. The skin looks muddy and flaky, and usually becomes dry. The muddy colour is the result of increasing anaemia, and also an increased amount of pigment in the skin, which also tans more in the sun than before. Sexual desire diminishes, and in men impotence is common. Movement and thought are slow. In children, bone pain and stunted growth may be particular problems.

As matters worsen more sinister symptoms may appear. The mouth has a persistent foul taste and food or, in smokers, cigarettes appear to change their flavour. The breath smells of ammonia and appetite diminishes, with nausea and sometimes vomiting. Cramps, especially at night, may be frequent and severe and interfere with fine work. Itching appears and may be severe, finally becoming an overwhelming torment, with scratch marks everywhere on the skin. Sleep is fitful and disturbed, with restlessness at night, jerking legs but drowsiness during the day, and the feet may burn and tingle. Finally, the patient may lapse into unconsciousness, have a fit, or develop severe pain in the chest indicating inflammation round the heart (pericarditis). Eyesight may become blurred, and transient blindness may even appear. Severe breathlessness is often present, with swelling of the ankles and bloating of the pallid, muddy face. Bleeding occurs at the corners of the mouth and from the nose, often with crusted sores which fail to heal. I hasten to add that fortunately this grim scenario is hardly ever played out to the end today, thanks to the availability of dialysis and transplantation (Chapters 6–10), and the aim is to start these treatments *before you get really ill*, which explains why your doctors may suggest treatments before you feel they are necessary, because at that point you may be feeling not too unwell, and it may be difficult to accept all the disturbance in your life that this brings.

These symptoms and signs of kidney failure are the complicated effect of the failure of the kidney to excrete poisonous substances, failure to regulate water and salt, and failure of the kidney's hormone production. We can now look a little more closely at how this happens.

Accumulation of toxic substances in the body fluids (failure of excretion)

As the kidneys' function fails the end-products of the body's metabolism, the clinker from the fire referred to in Chapter 1, accumulate to higher and higher levels in the blood (Chapter 2, Figure 8). It is this accumulation of poisonous rubbish in the body fluids which results in many of the symptoms just outlined, and finally, if unchecked, in death. The exact nature of these substances still is not entirely known. At least 150 different substances have been identified in normal urine, and in the blood of individuals with kidney failure, which might contribute to the toxicity of the state known as 'uraemia': that is, urine in the blood. One of these compounds is urea itself, which although the major product of the breakdown of nitrogen containing compounds in the human body, is not by itself very toxic. Much more toxic compounds have been identified, which affect cell function and the transmission of signals between and within cells, but it must be admitted that we cannot yet explain all the symptoms or signs you may get if you are uraemic.

Disorders of hormone production by the failing kidney

Vitamin D   As mentioned in Chapter 1, the kidney is the site of the final production of active vitamin D. As it fails, so production of vitamin D falls away. This results in a failure of calcium absorption from the bowel and failure of normal remodelling of bone. The effects depend upon whether the patient has stopped growing or not. If growth is still going on, then *rickets* appears, with defective growth, bowed legs, and broadening of the wrists and ankles. If growth has stopped then *osteomalacia* (soft bones in Greek) appears. This is mainly noticeable by pain in the pelvis and hips.

Erythropoietin (EPO)   Again as mentioned in Chapter 1, the kidney is the site of the production of the hormone which stimulates the bone marrow to make the red cells of the blood. This fails as the kidneys become scarred and contract. The smaller the kidneys, the lower the haemoglobin and red cell count in the blood. Thus patients with polycystic kidneys—which remain large—generally do not suffer from anaemia even when their kidneys have almost or completely stopped passing urine.

Renin   The production of renin from the kidneys is in general *increased* in kidney failure, which contributes to the salt retention and the high blood pressure. This is because the tissues of the scarred kidneys are receiving too little blood.

The adaptation of the kidney's function in renal failure (failure of regulation)

We described the kidney's normal functioning rather briefly in Chapter 1—now we can consider how the kidney adapts to progressive reduction in functioning kidney tissue. The aim of this section is to try and explain the very important point made in Figure 15—that is, as the kidney fails, although you can carry on much as before in normal circumstances, what is lost is *flexibility*. That is, the ability of your kidney to change its behaviour to meet changed circumstances.

To understand how this comes about is more difficult to explain in simple terms than the failure to excrete poisonous substances and the failure of the kidney to make vital hormones—indeed some doctors have difficulty understanding it! As the number of functioning nephrons declines in progressive kidney failure from the normal 2 million to only 100 000, each nephron is working not only normally but overtime; indeed, the surviving nephrons can be seen to increase in size if a failing kidney is examined down a microscope. As the numbers of units (nephrons) still functioning decrease, the balance of how each remaining tubule handles the filtered plasma water and salts must change. For example, the total amount of salt in the urine does not change much until the terminal stages of kidney failure. In a normal kidney, each tubule takes back 99.5 per cent of the salt reaching the tubules (Chapter 1); whereas in advanced renal failure only about 90 per cent is taken back, and 10 per cent allowed into the urine—that is, 20 times the normal amount. But there is a price to pay for this adaptation which permits one to live on one twentieth of normal kidney function. In health, the 0.5 per cent of sodium allowed into the urine in normal individuals can be varied to suit need (Chapter 1), but one problem in kidney failure is *loss of flexibility* (Figure 15). The kidney in advanced kidney failure may be putting out about the normal total amount of salt and water, but it *cannot vary this to meet the needs of day-to-day living*. In the case of phosphate, important for all tissues but especially bone, it is the level of parathyroid hormone (PTH) in the blood (see Chapter 1) which decreases the amount of phosphate taken back into the blood by the kidney tubule. The price of limiting the phosphate level in the blood by putting up the amount lost by each nephron is to raise the PTH level in the blood, and this brings about bone disease (see below). Without this reduction in the amount of phosphate reabsorbed, the individual with renal failure would turn, not like Lot's wife into a pillar of salt, but a pillar of chalk—or rather, calcium phosphate.

What are the signs of kidney failure?

Now we can go back and look at the many things that you or your doctor may notice going wrong as your kidneys fail, and try and explain them in terms of the loss of the kidney functions we have just described.

The heart

High blood pressure is commonly associated with chronic loss of kidney function, and the sufferer may go into heart failure, with a choking overload of water in the lungs. A more puzzling event is pericarditis, an inflammation of the sac around the heart, which is very characteristic of severe untreated kidney failure, and will often not go away unless dialysis is started. As already noted, high blood pressure may be without any symptoms and you do not know you have it. On the other hand, you may suffer from headaches, especially on getting up in the morning, disturbances in eyesight, breathlessness, or tightness in the chest.

The lungs

The uraemic patient is more prone to infection than normal, and in addition to the overload of water may suffer pneumonia in his already congested lungs.

The bowel

Loss of appetite and a foul taste in the mouth may be due to urea in the saliva and gastric juices. This is then broken down to ammonia which tastes unpleasant. Occasionally the lining of the bowel fails to repair itself properly and may lead to bloody diarrhoea.

The brain and nerves

The itching, burning, and numbness experienced by many uraemic subjects is probably associated with problems in the conduction of impulses up and down the nerves by the uraemic poisons in the tissue fluids. Perhaps the cramps also relate uraemic poisons in the tissue fluids, but may also result from loss of salt.

The bones and joints

Bone disease may appear, although this is not usually an early problem in adults; children and adolescents are principally affected, and along with this their growth is stunted. As just discussed, this bone disease has several causes: first, the kidney is the site of manufacture for the active form of vitamin D (see Chapter 1) and as the kidney is destroyed the levels of active vitamin D fall, and signs of vitamin D deficiency affect the bones, which differ according to whether you have stopped growing or not. Second, during uraemia there is a rise in the phosphate (phosphorus) in the blood, which causes the levels of the hormone produced by the parathyroid glands (PTH, see above) in the neck to rise during uraemia, which keeps the blood phosphate low, but also makes the bones lose calcium. Third, because the kidney cannot excrete acid normally, this is mopped up by the bones, which lose calcium in exchange for the acid. Children's and adolescents' bones are, of course, growing and making demands on all these systems, which probably explains why they have more trouble.

Joint trouble may also appear; this may resemble gout with an acutely inflamed, extremely painful single joint, but the substance involved is not often uric acid (even though the levels of uric acid in the blood are high in renal failure). Usually, it is a compound of calcium and phosphate (pyrophosphate) which appears because of the high phosphate level in the blood. This 'calcification' may also happen in the tissues around the joint, and this is equally painful!

The blood

Anaemia is one of the early and frequent features of kidney failure, as already noted. There are at least two main reasons for this. The first is that the production of the hormone which stimulates the marrow to make blood, erythropoietin (EPO, see Chapter 1), is reduced as the kidney is destroyed. This can be overcome by giving EPO (see treatment below) even though the marrow is also poisoned by uraemia. In addition to poor production, there is also an increased destruction of blood in the uraemic individual, because the red cells are stiffer and more fragile.

Endocrine glands

Loss of sexual desire and performance, impotence, and infertility with dis-appearance of the menstrual periods are common in uraemia. The complex interactions of hormones are disturbed in several directions in uraemia, some going up inappropriately, others becoming deficient.

The skin

The itching which plagues so many patients in uraemia—and on dialysis—is still a mystery. It appears likely that this is a sign of the nerve problem of uraemia, and like the tingling or burning in the feet, is a sensation in the absence of anything provoking it (paraesthesia), although this is still speculative. The dry, dull, flaky skin is the result of the failure of the skin to form a horny layer and have normal secretions. The pallor results from anaemia, and the pigment from both an increase in a hormone which controls pigment depositions which is normally broken down in the kidney. The pigments which normally colour urine are also present in excess in the blood, and this contributes to the muddy brown colour of uraemic skin.

How do we investigate chronic kidney failure?

In investigating someone who has been found to be in some degree of kidney failure, the doctor has several questions in mind.

How bad is the kidney failure?

Any patient who is identified—usually by blood tests—as having mild or severe impairment of kidney function will usually be referred to a specialist kidney unit for assessment.

The first steps are designed to assess the *degree* of chronic kidney failure. This involves, first, measurements of the substances in the blood which may be retained in kidney impairment—creatinine, urea, uric acid, phosphate— together with the blood electrolytes such as sodium, potassium, bicarbonate (see Chapter 2 for discussion). The blood calcium as well as phosphate will be examined to see if the expected depression of calcium in the presence of a high phosphate has occurred.

More precise measures of kidney failure can be obtained by assessing the glomerular filtration rate, or the clearance of creatinine by the kidneys from the blood (see Chapter 2). In addition, a 24-hour urine collection probably will be needed to estimate the loss of protein, especially if glomerulonephritis or other glomerular disease is the cause of the renal failure (see Chaptes 3 and 4).

What is the cause of the kidney failure? (see Chapters 3 and 4)

The second part of the investigation is concerned with trying to find the cause of the kidney failure, if this can be identified. Usually, the IVU X-ray or ultrasound of the kidneys will be done (Chapter 2), which may show the coarse scars of a reflux nephritis, in which case a cystogram (bladder X-ray) may be done (Chapter 2). If obstruction is seen on the ultrasound, then further tests to confirm this may be needed, such as special studies of pressures and flows within the urinary tract. If the bladder is suspected to be the site of the trouble, an examination of the bladder by cystoscopy may be performed (Chapter 2). If the kidneys are smooth in outline and the amount of proteinuria is large, so that a disease of the glomeruli is suspected, then a renal biopsy may be done (Chapter 2). Occasionally, an arteriogram may be needed to study the blood vessels if poor bloodflow from kidney blood vessel disease is suspected as a cause of the kidney failure, as may happen in older or diabetic subjects.

By this time it is usually clear what the problem may be, but in at least a quarter of patients—especially the elderly—there is no clear cause of the kidney failure, and both patient and doctor may have to accept that at least all immediately treatable causes of renal failure have been ruled out.

How fast is the kidney failure progressing?

Thereafter, the degree and progress of the kidney failure will be followed by regular measurements, principally of the blood creatinine and urea (Figure 16), whilst clinically a watch is kept on the blood pressure, if this is not already under treatment). The important fact will be how fast the measurements are changing, because these will usually reveal how things are going before you notice any change. Often it will be useful to plot out the results of the tests such as the plasma creatinine to reveal the course of the disease (Figure 16). Some patients may have conditions which progress slowly or not at all over many years—this may be the case after treatment of obstruction. Other conditions may progress very rapidly despite treatment, and take only a year or two to destroy the kidney to the point where dialysis of transplantation may be necessary. Obviously this point is likely to be reached earlier if the kidney is already badly damaged when it is first investigated, rather than approximately normal.

The tests may be done locally in your GP's surgery, at a local hospital, or at a special kidney unit. Generally all three may be involved, so as to limit visits to the specialist clinic, which may be a long way from home. On the other hand, special tests may be needed which can only be done there. In most

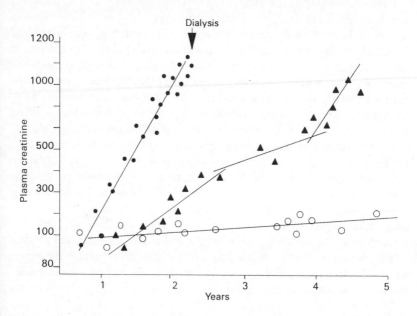

Figure 16 A plot of the creatinine level in the plasma in several patients with progressive kidney failure. Note that the figures have been plotted on a graph which does not have a linear scale on the left—it is a log scale. This 'straightens out' the rise in plasma creatinine concentrations shown in Figure 15, and allows better prediction of when end-stage kidney failure is likely to arrive. Note that in some patients the line even then is not straight, but can have sudden 'kinks' in it (black triangles) which prevent, or make difficult, any accurate prediction of how fast things will happen. A second patient, (open circles) has had almost no deterioration over five years, whilst a third (black dots) needed dialysis treatment for end-stage kidney failure in less than 2 years.

kidney units there is a special clinic for patients whose kidney failure is progressing, and who are expected to develop end-stage kidney failure.

The treatment of chronic kidney failure

Whilst watching we must obviously ask, what can be done to help you if you suffer from chronic loss of kidney function? Clearly the ultimate treatment may have to be some form of kidney replacement (see Chapters 6 to 10), but much can be done to help even if there is no specific treatment for your particular cause of kidney failure (Chapter 3).

First, *high blood pressure* must be identified and treated. This may not only relieve symptoms of breathlessness and chest pain, but may prolong the useful life of the kidneys (see Chapter 3 for details of treatment in blood pressure). Judicious use of diuretic drugs such as frusemide also helps lower the blood pressure. It is not clear yet whether some medicines rather than others are better for preservation of kidney function. However much information suggests that one group of drugs, the so-called ACE inhibitors (see Chapter 3) are better than any other form of blood pressure treatment in preserving kidney function.

Second, if anaemia is a severe problem, it can now be treated with EPO (erythropoietin) which disappears gradually as the kidneys are destroyed by whatever disease is affecting them. As noted above, diseases which lead to severe kidney destruction with very small kidneys tend to lead to more severe anaemia than those in which they remain large, such as polycystic kidney disease. The problems with EPO in patients with some kidney function are the same as those in patients already on dialysis—a tendency for the blood pressure to rise, which may be severe, and less commonly clots in major blood vessels. Of course the same high cost of EPO is present (see Chapter 6 for a fuller discussion of EPO).

Third, *diet* may help to make the best use of renal function, although the information on this point remains confusing, and different doctors place greater or lesser emphasis on the role of diet in the treatment of progressing kidney failure. The role of diet in the treatment of renal disease varies very much with the degree of renal failure. When the kidneys are functioning at a lowered level—say 50 per cent of normal, but the concentration of substances such as creatinine and urea is still relatively normal (Figure 16), the main dietary treatment that may be necessary is to avoid excessive salt intake in patients already with high blood pressure, or who are likely to develop it. The problem is to ask the patient to undertake a reduction in salt intake which can be maintained in the long-term; it is no use asking that salt be reduced to a level which cannot be tolerated and which will result in lapses within a few weeks at most. A combination of moderate salt restriction—say to about 4 g of salt per day in total, with no added salt at the table and an avoidance of very salty foods—together with some diuretic is best in the long run.

Whether limiting the protein (nitrogen) intake helps preserve kidney function remains a matter for debate, although it looks now as though any effect on prolonging kidney function, if present, is pretty small. The main problem is that many patients simply do not want to stick to rather restrictive diets in any case. Various doctors make different use of low protein diets in people with kidney failure at the moment, and as this is changing rapidly, I will not go into details on this here. In general a modest reduction in protein intake is useful, perhaps because of other reasons besides limiting nitrogen, as described in the next paragraph.

Fourth, to try and prevent *bone and joint problems* the control of blood phosphate levels is important. A low protein intake will also ensure a low phosphate intake, but agents to bind phosphate in the gut and prevent its absorption are important. These are usually calcium carbonate tablets, that is simple chalk, which also help raise the reduced level of calcium in the blood. Alternatively other calcium salts may be used, such as calcium acetate. Aluminium hydroxide gel (Aludrox, Basaljel), or aluminium hydroxide capsules (Alucaps) can also be used, but one must be aware of possible long-term toxic effects of the aluminium.

If bone problems do arise, or the tests suggest that they may be imminent, then treatment centres first around giving active forms of vitamin D. Vitamin D itself will not work, by and large, except in very big doses, because of the relative lack of kidneys to convert it into its native form (Chapter 1). Therefore the active form itself (calcitriol, sometimes called 1,25) or analogues such as alpha calcidol (Rocalcitrol, 1-alpha, alpha D) are used. In most patients these will produce an improvement, but in those with severe bone problems the main problem is not lack of active vitamin D, but overactivity of parathyroid glands. In that case, an operation to remove most or all of the parathyroid glands may be needed. This is a relatively small operation, and the scar on the neck is usually difficult to see afterwards, or can be covered by the collar or a necklace. If all the parathyroid glands are removed, as is common practice, then a small dose of vitamin D will be needed afterwards to help replace their absent function.

There is little that can be done to relieve the *itching* of chronic renal failure; keeping the skin moist with baby oil in the bath helps, but finally the only relief is relief of the uraemia. The *nausea and vomiting* of uraemia is helped by anti-emetic drugs, but again if severe and persistent will only respond to replacement therapy.

Occasional patients in advanced renal failure have problems with their blood *potassium* concentration. Too high a potassium level is bad for the heart, and may if extreme prove fatal. Usually, the kidney adapts by secreting far more potassium than usual from the tubules—up to 20 times the normal amount. Occasionally, however, the plasma potassium rises despite this, and the intake of potassium in the diet will be scrutinized to see if foods high in potassium are being taken. Some medicines, such as some blood pressure drugs like captopril and its relatives or beta-blockers (see Box 1), may increase the potassium, as will a few diuretics which are therefore usually avoided in patients with reduced kidney function. Thus the medicine chart must be looked at carefully if you have a potassium problem.

This brings up a particular problem which faces both patients with chronic kidney failure and the doctors looking after them: this is the fact that many medicines given for their treatment, or for incidental illnesses, may persist in the body at high concentrations because the kidney is one of the major routes for the removal of drugs and medicines from the body. If the agent is one which is principally got rid of through the kidney without an alternative route, then the dose may have to be reduced drastically, or the drug given on alternate days or even only twice or three times a week, that is much less frequently than usual. Prescribing for patients with kidney failure should always be done after careful thought as to the possible effects of the medicine in their particular circumstances.

Conclusions

Thus there is a great deal that can be done to help someone with kidney failure, even if the progress of the underlying disease cannot be stopped. During this period also, it will be possible to learn gradually about what is involved in the treatment of end-stage kidney failure by dialysis and transplantation, which is the next step for many patients. These topics are dealt with in the following chapters.

6 Artificial kidneys and dialysis

'After many early endeavours . . . an artificial kidney was constructed in cooperation with Mr H Th J Berk; an artificial kidney which is suitable for clinical use'

Willem ('Pim') Kolff (1911–   ) *New ways of treating uraemia*. 1947.

If your kidneys fail, fortunately it is possible to replace their function. One treatment for long-term kidney failure, a new kidney in the form of a kidney transplant, is dealt with in Chapter 8. This chapter concerns the methods of substituting for absent kidney function in other ways, usually called dialysis, which includes the use of an 'artificial kidney'. We are fortunate to have such treatments: a number of famous figures of the past, including Disraeli, Brunel, Jean Harlow, and possibly Mozart, died prematurely of renal failure.

The past 15 years have seen refinements in the use of the basic principles of dialysis, but the basic treatment is the same as that pioneered by Kolff, Scribner, and others (see Box 3). The external plastic shunt has, for long-term dialysis, been all but replaced by internal junctions (fistulae) made by joining arteries and veins directly, introduced in 1967 by doctors in New York. The dialysers ('artificial kidneys') are now much smaller, and usually disposable after one or a few uses. Portable machines are available, but a practical wearable machine is not yet with us (see Chapter 11). New membranes have been introduced to replace those which are essentially the same as those used in Baltimore by Abel and his colleagues in 1913, and new techniques can remove excess fluid much more easily from the body. But dialysis is performed today in the same fundamental way as it was 80 years ago.

Thus, for the formerly untreatable condition of irreversible kidney failure we now have three alternative forms of treatment: haemodialysis, CAPD, or transplantation. This chapter deals with haemodialysis, Chapter 7 with CAPD, and Chapter 8 with transplantation.

What does going on to dialysis mean for me?

If you are to be started on to haemodialysis, you will often know in advance, and have been prepared to some extent during attendance at the special clinic for such patients in the local kidney unit (see Chapter 5); you may already have had a *fistula* (see below) for blood access placed in an arm in preparation for beginning dialysis. Some unlucky patients, however, come to hospital already in need of dialysis and may have to be treated immediately. Sometimes, peritoneal dialysis (Chapter 7) will be started first while their arm fistula matures. Sometimes, a *neck line* (see below) will be put in as well as a fistula, for use only until the fistula is ready.

Either way, the impact of starting dialysis is considerable! It involves the whole family, and the social workers, nurses, and doctors will need to talk to your partner as well, since all will be anxious at this time. Knowing what to expect is half the battle, and this is the object of this chapter. The impact of dialysis in terms of lost time may be great, since travelling time must be added to the treatment time, and dialysis to begin with will be during the daytime; a recovery period after each dialysis may be necessary until the system has adjusted to the procedure. This is bound to result in time off work and financial worries may add to all the other anxieties; most employers are sympathetic, but the self-employed face special problems. A chat with someone who has already had experience of dialysis and other treatments for renal failure can be a great help; after all, they know what it is like whilst the doctors and nurses only see it from the outside. Patients' associations, local or national, are a great help (see the list in Appendix 2). Children and their parents, of course, face special anxieties.

Even if expecting it, anyone is bound to find adjusting to life on dialysis difficult. On the other hand, for some it comes as a relief after a period in limbo, during which no plans can be made for the future. Dietary needs will change, but one main problem on dialysis is *limiting fluid intake*. How much fluid can be taken very much depends on whether high blood pressure is present, and how much urine your kidneys are still passing. Both may gradually diminish over the first few months, and whilst easier blood pressure is good news, loss of some urine output may result in a tightening of restriction on water intake. Most patients will only be able to take about 500 ml (one pint) of fluid per day.

To begin with, it is likely that you may be unwell at the end of each dialysis, partly because tremendous changes are occurring in the composition of body fluids and partly because your circulation is encountering a number of foreign materials for the first time. This is not always the case, and anyway it is usual for well-being to improve after the first week. Then a plan must be made for the future. Nowadays, haemodialysis, CAPD, and transplantation are seen everywhere as *fully integrated approaches* to end-stage kidney failure, rather than competing treatments, and this is discussed later in Chapter 10.

Box 3   A little history: how do artificial kidneys work?

The story of the introduction of the artificial kidney is a dramatic one, depending upon the far-sightedness and even obstinacy of a few pioneers. Many people know how a Dutchman, Willem (Pim) Kolff constructed the first practical artificial kidney in the Netherlands in the depths of the Second World War, and showed that it could save the lives of people in temporary kidney failure. However, to understand where we are today it is useful to review in brief what has gone before.

The first understanding of the problem rests on the discovery in the nineteenth century by the Scottish chemist, Robert Graham, of the rules governing the movement of substance dissolved in water. This process of 'diffusion' of dissolved substances from places with a high concentration to areas of low concentration, so that eventually the concentration equalized everywhere is the basis of substituting renal function by the artificial kidney or other forms of dialysis. Graham also studied what happened if membranes were placed between two solutions with a high and low concentration of solutes, and showed that some membranes would let through small molecules, whereas they did not permit the passage of larger ones. These 'semipermeable' membranes are crucial components in all forms of *dialysis*—the name Graham gave to this process. In Greek, it means disintegration, but is now universally used to mean the process of separation by diffusion across membranes, such as the artificial kidney performs.

The first 'artificial kidney' used to perform dialysis on blood haemodialysis was built and used surprisingly early by Drs Abel, Rowntree, and Turner in Baltimore in the USA in 1913. They had to prepare their own membranes out of collodion tubes, but came up with a startlingly modern design for their 'kidney' similar in principle to those used today. One problem was that they had to prevent the blood of dogs they dialysed from clotting. For this they used a crude extract of leeches, which had to be prepared fresh for each run of the machine. The use of dialysis in humans was brought nearer by the introduction of the substance *heparin*, which will also prevent blood-clotting, in 1926. This is a safe anticoagulant with a brief action which can be injected repeatedly, and is still the mainstay of contemporary dialysis.

Although a German, Haas, did some dialyses in patients (including some in kidney failure) in the 1920s, using a kidney based on that of Abel and his colleagues, two men are chiefly responsible for the use of the artificial kidney: Pim Kolff in Holland and Nils Alwall in Sweden, working independently during and just after World War II. They explored designs of kidney different from those explored previously by the Americans, and in particular Kolff pioneered the 'coil' design which was used until recently.

The advantages of using the 'artificial kidney' for temporary kidney failure became recognized rather slowly, but by 1960 treatment of acute, reversible renal failure by temporary dialysis was routine in many centres round the world. The problem was how to get blood out of the patient repeatedly to pass through the machine and back into the body. At that time, cannulas made of glass or metal put into blood vessels which had to be cut across only lasted a short while, and the vessels were destroyed in the process. Obviously, dialysis could only be performed for a few days, or weeks at most. Then, in 1960, Belding Scribner (know to everyone as 'Scrib') a physician, and Wayne Quinton, an engineer, and their associates in Seattle introduced a new cannula which lasted for months or even years. It was made of what were then new plastics (PTFE (Teflon R)) and silicone rubber) with which the blood did not react. Scribner and his associates tested the effects of repeated dialysis on patients with irreversible kidney failure, and then realized that they became better and could leave hospital, returning only for their dialysis treatment. Plastic tubing was introduced about the same time, and could be used to connect the patient's cannulas to the dialyser which also made repeated dialysis treatment possible. It is now difficult to realize what dialysis was like using crude rubber tubing sterilized before each session. Dialysers which could be re-used were built, and within only two or three years, the first patients were using them regularly at home to dialyse themselves. Stanley Shaldon, in the United Kingdom, was the first to realize how successful home dialysis could be for selected patients.

Let us suppose that the decision is made, after discussion with you and your family (see Chapter 10), that long-term haemodialysis will be the choice for first treatment.

What does haemodialysis involve?

If you are going to start dialysis, naturally you will want to know something about what is going on. First, let us go over the components of the machinery that you will be connected to, and then come back to what dialysis involves for you.

The principles of haemodialysis are discussed in Box 3. Figures 17 and 18 show in diagrammatic form a dialysis circuit. First, *blood* is taken out of the body, usually from blood vessels in an arm (see below) and is treated with an *anticoagulant* to prevent it clotting when in contact with the plastics and surfaces outside the body. Then the blood is pumped into a *dialyser* where it passes over semipermeable membranes, usually made of cellulose even today, through which an exchange of dissolved substances (dialysis) takes place. The exchange occurs across the membrane into and from a solution (*dialysate*), the

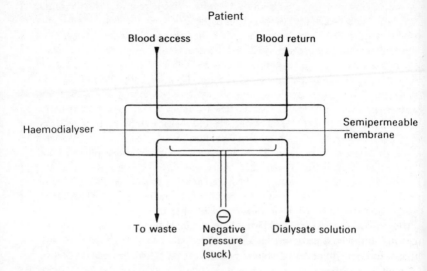

Figure 17 The basic haemodialysis circuit, or 'artificial kidney'. See text for discussion.

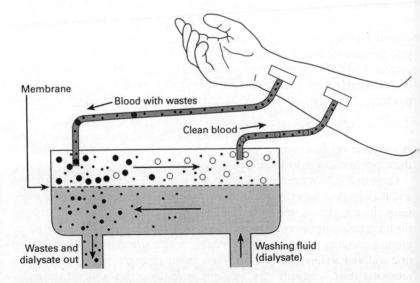

Figure 18 The exchanges that take place between the blood and the dialysate fluid within the artificial kidney during dialysis. See text for further discussion.

composition of which can be determined by those doing the dialysis. In general, the make-up of this fluid approximates to an ideal solution of the body's salts dissolved in water. It need not be sterile because the membrane is too thick to allow bacteria through, although some products from dead bacteria can penetrate and cause problems on occasion. The dialysis solution does not, however, contain any of the poisonous products of metabolism such as urea, creatinine, and the other substances known to accumulate in patients with renal failure. It will be low in potassium, which tends to accumulate, and contains no phosphate, which is at the same time an essential fuel but also a waste product, and which also accumulates in kidney failure.

The blood flows continuously around through the dialyser during the dialysis session which usually lasts four hours or a little less, and the fresh fluid is passed through it on the other side of the membrane continuously, so that a high gradient of the toxic substances is always present between the blood, and their passage out of the blood is made more rapid. Meanwhile, no bacteria can get in, and no red cells, white cells, or proteins from the blood can pass out through the membrane. The blood returning from the dialyser is almost devoid of toxic substances accumulated in kidney failure, but, of course, blood only forms a small part of the body fluids, all of which are full of the same materials. Thus, the 'cleaned' blood picks up more uraemic poisons from the water outside the cells—the extracellular 'soup' (see Chapter 1), and then returns to the dialyser to discharge them. In turn, the water outside the cells loses urea, creatinine, etc. and can in turn allow diffusion of these substances out of the cells themselves. In fact, *this exchange out of the cells, over which we have no control*, is the slowest exchange, and limits the speed with which dialysis can be performed. Also it goes on long after you have disconnected from the machine. Thus, the exchange in the dialyser is only one of several in a series:

dialysate ⇌ blood ⇌ extracellular water ⇌ water within cells

A molecule of (for example) urea from inside a cell must pass through all of these before it can be lost from the body.

Large molecules move more slowly down this gradient than small molecules, and may be held up more at the membrane. For example, uric acid is three times the size of urea, and correspondingly dialyses out more slowly. Some of the main toxic substances in uraemia seem to be even bigger—they fall into the group sometimes called 'middle molecules' with a size up to 10 times that of uric acid, and 30 times that of urea. Thus, haemodialysis is not very efficient at removing them, and this may account for its failure to restore patients to complete health.

Another problem arises, and that is how to remove *water*. Whilst in theory it is possible to take in no more water than is lost by the bowel and in sweat or in the breath, in practice this is almost impossible; most foods contain a great deal of water. For example, meat is 70 per cent water, and a cucumber or a melon 98 per cent water. Even if your fluid intake is limited to an intake of 500 ml (one pint) a day, and you stick to it, your total intake will be more than a litre (two to two and a half pints). If dialysis is done every second or third day, you can easily see that at least 1.5 litres of water, maybe more will have to be removed. How is this achieved?

Most dialysers remove water by a form of suction, called *ultrafiltration*. This involves the bulk passage of water (and its dissolved salts) across the membrane, and it can be achieved very easily. What is required is to bring a *pressure gradient* across the membrane. Already, the pump pushing the blood into the dialyser is generating some pressure, and this can be increased either by lowering the pressure on the other side of the dialysis membrane using another pump (this is usually called 'suck' by those doing dialysis); equally, the outflow of blood from the dialyser can be restricted by a gateclip on the tubing and this raises the pressure in the blood compartment, because the pressure of the blood pump meets resistance and the pressure rises to overcome it and keep blood-flow constant. Ultrafiltration can be done during the dialysis, or separately before dialysis begins which some patients find more gentle.

Let's look at each component of the system in a little more detail.

How does blood get to the dialyser?

This has very considerable impact on you, the patient, since reliable, pain-free access to the dialyser is crucial in allowing smooth treatment free of anxiety. The commonest access in use for long-term haemodialysis is using an A–V (*arterio–venous*) *fistula* (Figure 19 and Plate 15). For this a small operation is done, usually in the wrist of the nondominant arm (left for the majority of right-handed people). The radial artery is joined, usually side to side at the wrist so that the vein back up the arm increases in size and develops a thicker wall.

You will notice that after the fistula has been formed that you can feel a buzzing over it, which is a sign that the fistula is working well. If your fistula stops buzzing, it may be a sign that it has clotted, and you should let the unit know if this happens. Don't let anyone take blood from, or put an infusion into your fistula arm—your fistula is precious. Don't wear anything tight on the fistula arm either, which might obstruct the flow of blood back up the fistula.

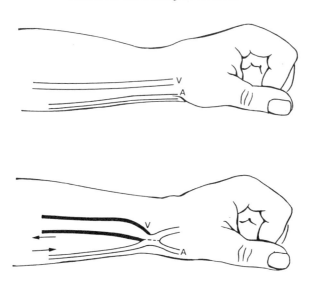

Figure 19 An arteriovenous fistula. The artery (A) and vein (B) at the wrist are brought together by a surgical operation. The blood flows at arterial pressure into the vein, which dilates and develops a thickened wall (sometimes it is necessary to tie off the distal part of the vein to the hand; this is not shown in the diagram). This enlarged artery-like vein can then be needled to provide blood to and receive blood from the dialyser.

This enlarged vein (Plate 15 (top)) is then needled (Plate 15 (bottom)) at each dialysis to provide access to the bloodstream, first to withdraw blood and then to return it after it has passed through the dialyser. Usually, the A (arterial, taking) needle is placed face downstream nearer the fistula, and the V (venous, return) needle further up the arm. Fistulas can also be made further up the arm, at the elbow.

In fact only one needle is absolutely necessary, which can be used alternately every few seconds to give and to take blood. This is referred to as a 'single-needle' system and is being used more and more nowadays. This has the advantage of only requiring one needle, but sometimes dialysis is less efficient because blood recirculates and is dialysed over and over, rather than returning to mix in the rest of the bodyd, which it must if dialysis is to be efficient.

Needles and needling Most people are understandably afraid of either having needles stuck into them, or doing it themselves. In fact, puncture of a fistula is relatively painless, since very sharp thin wall needles covered with silicone to prevent clotting are used. Many patients feel that injecting local anaesthetic is more painful than inserting the needle itself, but local anaesthetic gel rubbed on the skin helps a lot for those who need it.

The first few punctures on a new fistula are often more difficult than later, and bruising is more likely, so don't worry! However things usually get better very quickly, as the fistula thickens up and some scar tissue forms. To begin with also one has to find where the best places are on the fistula for taking blood, and for giving it back. This can take time also. Once the best places are established, it is important not to take the blood from precisely the same spot, but to 'walk' the needles up and down the fistula over a centimetre or two, so that the fistula wall doesn't get weakened and cause 'blow-out' with a bulge in the wall which may need to be repaired.

During the dialysis the needles are strapped to the arm for safety and towards the end of dialysis the pump giving the anticoagulant (heparin) is usually switched off early, then at the end a dose of a substance to neutralize the heparin, called protamine, is sometimes given to minimize bleeding from the puncture sites when the needles are taken out.

Training to needle yourself depends on a number of things: how good your eyesight is, how good you are with your hands—anyone with shaky hands or bad arthritis may find it difficult. The main obstacle, however, is fear of the needle and the process—so called 'needle phobia'. Everyone has this to a certain extent, but for some people it is an overwhelming problem and if they are to have dialysis they may need help from a psychologist, who will use one of several techniques to diminish this fear.

Complications of fistulas   Immediately after the fistula has been made, the hand may get too little bloodflow, because the blood is diverted into the vein and rushes back up the arm to the heart. This results in cold painful fingers or hand. Often this improves but may result in the fistula having to be refashioned or even reversed. This complication is much commoner in older patients with blood vessel disease, and in diabetics. On the other hand, if the fistula is too big, too much blood may flow down the vein into the hand, which becomes hot and swells up sometimes with pain. Again this may need correction. Sometimes the fistula is too small, and clots off completely, and so is not useable. In that case a new one must be fashioned.

In general, in the long term fistulas once established give few problems. Some women, and a few men, find them too unsightly to tolerate, or keep them covered at all times. 'Blow outs' at weak points in the wall have been mentioned, and the needle site can become infected so that the entry point has to be changed, or the fistula rested until the infection has been treated by antibiotics.

Occasionally, fistulas may clot off even when running well, usually in association with being too 'dry' after dialysis, that is too much fluid has been removed during the dialysis (see below) so that the blood pressure drops too low and the bloodflow through the fistula is very small.

Artificial fistulae

Some people have difficulty in keeping an open fistula; they clot it off, despite the use of anticlotting drugs. Often they are the ones with the highest haemoglobin who are fittest! In such patients, alternative means of access may be necessary, and some kidney units now use them as a routine. The commonest involves the use of artificial substances to sew in an artery–vein connection under the skin; an artery–artery connection is also useful. The material used is most commonly Goretex (R) which is made of the same PTFE (Teflon (R)) used in the external plastic shunt, but this time in woven form. It is now familiar as a material for anoraks and tents, but here it is woven into a tube, which is cut to the right length and sewn in either as a loop, or a bridge, depending on whether the arm has been operated on before (Figure 20).

Other materials can be used, such as knitted Dacron (R), but clot more readily; more promising are 'natural' materials such as the patient's own vein,

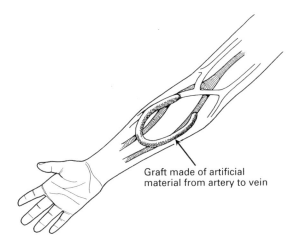

Graft made of artificial
material from artery to vein

Figure 20 A diagram of a graft between an artery and a vein in the forearm, to be used as access for taking and returning blood from the dialyser. The tube is sewn into place and, unlike the natural fistula in Figure 19 and Plate 15, can usually be used almost immediately.

taken usually from the leg; or dried and sterilized animal vessels (usually arteries), which are dead, but act as a framework for the body to coat with its own cells. Veins from the birthcord of babies (which is usually thrown away with the afterbirth) have been tried also. You can see that the ideal solution has not yet been found by the variety of materials being tried!

'Neck lines': (Subclavian/jugular vein catheters)

Fistulas cannot be used immediately—usually one has to wait 2–6 weeks before the veins have enlarged and thickened enough to be needled. What if you need dialysis straight away? Use has been made of temporary silastic cannulas put into the large veins in the upper chest (Figure 21 and Plate 16). They can also be put into the jugular vein in the side of the neck (Plate 17). Most of these cannulas have a double channel, others are used like a single needle. They can be put in quickly using local anaesthetic, and can be left for days or weeks. If placed in the large vein in the chest leading from the arm to the heart (the subclavian vein) they can be used for months if put in in an operating room under full sterile conditions; for this a general anaesthetic may be needed. In

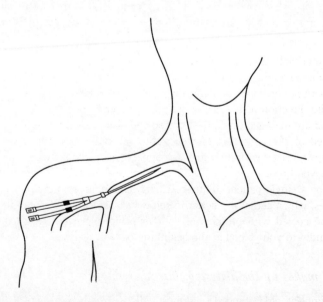

Figure 21 A diagram of a subclavian line. The double lumen catheter for taking and returning blood is passed round a wire through the skin into the large vein leading into the heart from the arm—the subclavian vein.

this type of procedure, sometimes a long-dwelling catheter called a Hickman catheter is used.

The principal problem with subclavian vein catheters (Figure 21 and Plate 16) is infection on the end lying in the blood stream, and scarring of the vein where the tip of the catheter lies, so that when it is taken out blood has difficulty getting past, and a fistula made in the arm on that side may be difficult to use because of high pressure. These narrowings, or stenoses as they are called, may need to be dilated by a balloon catheter passed up the arm to lower the pressure during dialysis.

What are dialysers like? (Figure 22)

There have been many variations in design, but today the main variety used is the *hollow fibre dialyser* (Figure 22(a)), in which the blood is passed through thousands of minute hollow fibres of membrane, round which the dialysate flows in the opposite direction.

In some units *flatbed dialysers* (Figure 22(b)) are used. In these, a stack of membranes and spaces for dialysis fluid (dialysate) are arranged in a sandwich. This design is used also for dialysers and filters for use in temporary (acute) kidney failure.

Only of historical interest now is the *coil dialyser*, in which the membrane is a long flat bag wound in a spiral coil through which the dialysate is pumped, usually at right angles. This type of dialyser was used as standard for acute reversible kidney failure for 20 years up to 1970.

In both hollow fibre and flatbed types of dialyser, blood is made to flow in the opposite direction to the dialysate to improve efficiency.

Most are manufactured pre-sterilized and disposable, and are intended to be disposed of after one use. However they are often re-sterilized and re-used (perhaps together with their lines to connect you to the dialyser) after sterilization, several times, and often are because of cost, up to 10 times or more, but only for a single patient. Thus you may have your own dialyser for several dialyses, which actually is better in some ways, since the inside of the dialyser become coated with proteins of your own blood plasma, and makes it less unfriendly to your blood at the beginning of each dialysis.

What makes up the dialysing fluid (dialysate)?

The simplest, old-fashioned—but most tedious—method to make dialysate is to add salts to a volume of water in a tank, and mix them by hand. A large volume is needed for dialysis—the human body contains about 45 litres (10 gallons) of

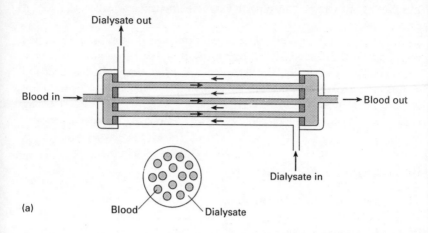

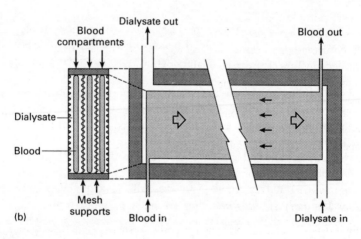

Figure 22 Diagrams of two types of dialyses (artificial kidneys). (a) The *hollow fibre kidney* consists of a large number of very fine tubes made of semipermeable cellulose membrane, through which blood passes and exchanges with a stream of dialysate fluid which is passing in the opposite direction and then passes to waste. Only a few tubes are shown, but in the actual artificial kidney many thousands are used. This is the commonest type of kidney used today. (b) The *flatbed (or plate) dialyser* employs a series of flat blood compartments with membranes separating the blood from the dialysis fluid, which, as in the hollow fibre kidney, is pumped in the opposite direction to the blood-flow to increase the efficiency of the system. The blood compartments alternate with supports which both contain the blood compartment, keeping it flat and thin, and also allow the dialysis fluid to pass.

water (Chapter 1), and about 100–500 litres (25–125 gallons) of dialysate are required; hence if all dialysis is in a tank, it has to be fairly large! The usual method used today is more expensive, but much more convenient (Plate 18). This is a pumped system in which a concentrated solution is mixed automatically with water by a blending pump, heated up to blood temperature, checked for composition, and fed into the dialyser. A concentrate can be fed from a small tank at about 30–40 times the final concentration to mix with an appropriate amount of water.

Although the dialysate water does not have to be sterile, it must be pure, and not contain too much calcium or aluminium. Most tap-water in the southern half of the UK already contains too much calcium, so that *softened* water must be used. In addition, there are many other contaminants even in 'pure' tap-water which may cause harm if accumulated in the body and units may employ water purified by *de-ionization* using a resin column which takes out all charged molecules; or by RO (*reverse osmosis*), a filtration system used on an industrial scale to make drinking water out of sea water in arid countries.

Obviously, if the water already used for a dialysis could be treated in turn to remove the toxic products dialysed out of the blood of the patient, then a very much smaller amount of dialysate could be used. This in turn would make dialysis more easy and more portable. Such a system is (the REDY (R)), which uses only 4 litres (8 pints) of dialysate, which is purified and re-used again and again by a column through which the dialysate passes. This however adds considerably to the cost of each dialysis, although it is very convenient where water supplies are limited or impure, and for holidays.

What does the dialysis 'machine' do? Monitoring of dialysis

Especially if dialysis is being performed at home, perhaps at night (see below), then it must be completely safe. To ensure this, a number of automatic checks must be made in the system by the monitoring system (Plate 18).

(1) That the dialyser is not *leaking blood* into the dialysate. The membranes are very thin (down to 10 μm, or 1/2500 inch) and rupture could lead to blood loss.

(2) That no *bubbles* are returning into you in the venous line. The circuit incorporates a 'bubble trap' but this can fill up with foam (the reasons for bubbling in the circuit are complicated and cannot be gone into here) and a monitor is needed on the bubble trap (BT in Plate 18), usually based on the amount of light from a bulb that can get through.

(3) That the *temperature* of the dialysate is just above blood temperature, so that you don't steadily cool during the procedure, or overheat.

(4) That the *composition* of the dialysate is accurate. This is usually measured as a total electrical conductivity, since the concentrate is constant and is prechecked.

(5) That the *amount* of 'suck' (negative pressure) is appropriate so the right amount of fluid will be lost during the dialysis session.

(6) That the *blood pressure* on the arterial, giving, and venous, returning, side of the circuit are appropriate.

Many of these functions are controlled by a microchip in modern monitoring systems. Thus, the dialysis 'machine' on to which the actual dialyser (Plate 18) is clamped incorporates not only pumps, tanks, and lines, but also a *monitoring console* which is usually equipped with a 'fail-safe' system, which stops the dialysate and blood pump if an alarm state is indicated in any of the above systems, and gives an audible and a visual signal that all is not well. It also signals if the electricity or water supply has failed. Dialysis can sometimes be a rather noisy procedure!

There are many different systems on the market, which usually incorporate the preparation of dialysate and monitoring systems. Most now incorporate a small microchip computer so that at the beginning of dialysis you can 'dial in' the weight loss you would like, and refinements such as checking on the blood flow from your fistula through the dialyser—which is an important factor in how effective the dialysis session will be (see below).

What is a dialysis like?

Obviously the only way to know is to experience one, or at least to visit the dialysis unit before you start dialysis. This is always useful because not only can you see what the machinery is like and what goes on, but you can talk to other patients who are already doing what you are about to begin. However a brief description of the whole business may be useful.

Almost everyone begins dialysis within a central unit, whether later they may be dialysing in a smaller satellite unit or at home (see below). This means if you are an out-patient arriving at the dialysis unit in enough time to get settled before your scheduled dialysis time. Transport to the unit can be a real difficulty, especially if you are not well to begin with, whether it is problems with hospital transport not arriving on time, catching the right train, or difficulties in parking your car. This is usually worse in big city centres.

Once at the dialysis unit, your blood pressure will be checked, standing and lying, and your weight will be measured. This allows the staff to judge how much fluid you have gained since the dialysis. Maybe they will look at your neck to see the veins there, look at your ankles, and listen to your chest to see how much water there is in them, to help with this assessment. After a brief wait you will be sat down in a rather special reclining chair for the dialysis. Then the needles must be put in. Each needle carries on it a syringe full of salt solution with heparin in it to prevent clotting. Local anaesthetic is injected or rubbed in at the site to be punctured and the needle eased into the fistula through the skin. Usually the needle which will be taking the blood is labelled with red and the needle which will give the blood back with blue; the first is often called the arterial, or A needle, and the latter the venous or V needle.

Before you arrived, the unit staff will have prepared your machine for use. There are many types of machine, so a detailed description is not possible. However on the machine, with its plastic tubing attached, will be the actual dialyser. This is a surprisingly small tube sitting in clamps on the 'kidney machine', whose components were described above. The lines from the needles are connected to the lines, the clamp on the A line removed and the bloodpump started. You will see the blood enter the dialyser, colour it red and then flow back into the V line, whilst the salt solution from the inside of the dialyser runs to waste. Then the V line is connected to the V needle and the circuit can start running. The needles are taped to your arm for safety during the dialysis.

The length of dialysis, dose of heparin, and amount of pressure for fluid removal will have been decided by the unit staff beforehand to suit your individual needs. During the dialysis there is usually little for you to do except read, study, chat, knit, sleep, or watch the television. Occasionally alarms may go off (see above) and you or the staff will need to make adjustments to the machine.

Usually you will feel well during the dialysis, but if a large amount of fluid has to be removed you may suffer from painful cramps—a good reason for not putting on the weight in the first place! Some people get backache during dialysis for reasons that are not clear. If your blood pressure drops too low, you may feel 'woozy' and you will need to have some saline solution infused. Some people who have heart trouble may experience chest pain (angina) during dialysis, and the staff need to know about this. Usually more gentle dialysis, or EPO to raise your level of haemoglobin will make this better.

A little while before the end of the dialysis, the heparin pump will be shut off. Then when it is time to stop, obviously the dialyser is full of your blood, which is precious. Thus it will need to be washed back into you through the V (venous) needle into your arm, using the pump. Thus the A line is clamped, separated, or cut and connected with a salt (saline) solution, which is pumped into the dialyser so that the blood goes back up your arm. Then both lines can be clamped and the needles removed. You will need to press for a while on the punctures to stop them bleeding. Before you go home, your weight will be checked to see how much fluid you lost whilst on the machine, and your blood pressure checked again lying and standing to see the effect on your circulation.

How you feel immediately after dialysis varies from person to person. Some feel fine, but others feel very 'washed out' especially if they had gained a lot of weight and had therefore to lose a great deal (more than 2 kg for example).

How often and for how long must I dialyse?

Usually patients on haemodialysis will need three sessions each week of about 4 hours; some a little less, some a little more, largely depending on how big they are. Of course there is preparation and getting on to the machine before, and coming off and clearing up after, so that it takes about six hours altogether.

Nowadays it is usual to assess each patient carefully according to their sex, age, body size, amount of fat, and the figures in their blood and the blood flow which can be obtained through their fistula, and prescribe an individual amount of dialysis to suit each person at each time. One of the calculations which is done to assess this is called the Kt/V (pronounced kay tee over vee) which you may hear mentioned. All patients should have enough dialysis to ensure a Kt/V of more than about 1.2, and many doctors feel that 1.3 or more is better. From time to time you will be asked to provide a 24-hour urine collection so the unit staff can measure what little function is left in your own kidneys. Thus, dialysis schedules vary somewhat from patient to patient, some getting off dialysis earlier. It is important *not* to cut corners and try and reduce dialysis hours, since usually the doctors will have prescribed only just a little more dialysis than is needed, to try and let you off the machine as soon as possible, and cutting it further may result in your not having enough dialysis.

Some units dialyse some smaller patients only twice a week, but many doctors are not happy that this can provide enough dialysis for the best of health. Certainly, each dialysis session needs to be longer if only two dialyses per week are performed.

Where can I dialyse?

There are several options for haemodialysis. First, you can travel three times a week to a *dialysis centre*, usually in a hospital, where you will have dialysis together with a dozen other patients. Usually in these circumstances you may take little part in the procedure to begin with, but as you become confident you may well want to put your own needle in, and to run your own dialysis under supervision of the dialysis unit staff. The advantage of centre dialysis is that you don't have to worry about the details of the dialysis if you don't want to. The disadvantages are that you have to travel to the centre—which may be some distance, and difficult if you have to use a hospital car or an ambulance— and that you cannot always have your dialysis when you would like it.

In a *limited care or satellite unit*, you will usually have to be able to supervise your own dialysis to some extent, since staff are often limited in number and may not be fully trained to run a dialysis. The advantage of the limited care or satellite unit is that it is often nearer your home. Usually fitter and more capable patients will transfer to a satellite unit if one is available nearer their homes. These need not be in a hospital (although some are), but may be a converted house or a purpose built facility. Usually these are smaller than dialysis units and three or four patients dialyse at the same time.

Finally, you may wish to do *home haemodialysis*. For this you will need extensive training to be completely self-sufficient. It goes without saying that to have home dialysis you have to have a home. Most units would also prefer that there is some other supporting partner, who can deal with emergencies, at home. This can be a problem, especially if they eventually feel they no longer wish to play this role. It also excludes most young unmarried people living alone, and ties adolescents down into the family home if the parents are to provide the support.

The degree of interference with the home for home dialysis varies with different units' philosophies of how home dialysis should be conducted. Some prefer a separate room, others will use the usual bedroom or sitting room. Both have psychological and physical advantages. Space for storing the disposable lines, fluids, drugs, etc. will always be required. Finally, the machine, the dialyser, the water softener, de-ionizer, or RO machine must be accommodated. All this needs space, and in some houses this just cannot be found. Sometimes a portable home can be put in a garden; it may even be necessary to rehouse a family to achieve successful home dialysis, and in many cities the local council may have flats or houses already converted for dialysis which become available from time to time—for example if someone who has a successful transplant moves away.

Training for home haemodialysis varies in length; usually, the house is not ready by the time training is complete. Most units prefer six weeks' training with the supporting person coming for the last two weeks, but often longer will be required; some people are fast learners, others require more time but may well be safer and better at it in the end. The important point is to make you self-reliant, but most pairs of partners will work out patterns of responsibility later which may differ from what the unit aims for!

Once established, regular deliveries of supplies come from the supporting unit. Technicians, nurses, social workers, and doctors are available for support in the parent unit, and a telephone at home is essential.

The advantages of home dialysis are the independence and self-confidence you have together with the ability to dialyse on a schedule that suits your own weekly pattern of life. Many patients dialyse two evenings a week with another session at the weekend; others prefer three overnight sessions a week. Home dialysis is a good deal cheaper than centre dialysis. The disadvantages of home dialysis are the strain imposed on the family, and the time in preparing the machine which is provided ready in the dialysis unit.

Dialysing *on holiday* obviously presents problems, but these can be overcome since many units in the UK and overseas will accept patients for dialysis. Usually the financial arrangements can be covered within the budget of the unit. Many units have a holiday dialysis facility of their own, and the British Kidney Patients' Association (see Appendix 2) has holiday units in the UK and abroad. Alternatively, if you are home trained you may be able to have training to take a mobile unit such as a REDY with you on holiday.

What medicines will I need to take whilst on haemodialysis?

In general the only medicines that will be needed will be:

(i)   *Iron*, because it is absorbed poorly if you are uraemic.

(ii) *Vitamins*, because some of them are dialysed out by the dialyser, including folic acid which is often given as a separate tablet. However, if you are eating a well-balanced diet containing enough vitamins these may not be necessary.

(iii) *Phosphate binders*. Medicines take phosphate out of your blood (*phosphate binders*), such as calcium carbonate (chalk) or aluminium hydroxide, will usually be necessary since if you eat enough protein to keep your muscles and other tissues healthy, then you will at the same time be taking in phosphate.

(iv) If your bones are giving problems (see Chapter 5) then it may be necessary to take a small dose of a *vitamin D* preparation such as calcitriol

(1,25) or alpha calcidol(1-alpha) to protect your bones, but unfortunately this often leads to the calcium level in the blood going too high.

(v) If you have high blood pressure despite dialysis—which is quite common with the short dialysis schedules used today—then you may need tablets to help lower your blood pressure. Details of the various medicines used for this are given in Chapter 4.

(vi) EPO, if your haemoglobin remains low despite adequate dialysis.

(vii) *Laxatives*, if you are constipated; this can be a problem for dialysis patients because of their lack of exercise and low fluid intake. Don't buy them yourself from the chemist, because some are not suitable for someone without kidneys; ask the staff of the unit about this problem.

(viii) Obviously also, diabetics will need to continue their insulin injections, or tablets to control their diabetes. Some anti-diabetic tablets are unsuitable for people in kidney failure, and may have to be changed to ones which are got rid of by the liver rather than the kidneys. Similarly, for some other diseases which cause kidney failure, the treatment for these may have to be continued whilst on dialysis.

How important is diet in haemodialysis?

Diet is *extremely* important for patients on dialysis. First, fluid restriction has already been mentioned. You will be given a 'target' or 'dry' weight to try and achieve at the end of each dialysis, and to hold as best you can until the next one. Usually your intake will be the equivalent of the volume of urine you pass, plus about 2½ ordinary cups (500 ml).

It is important to take in enough protein to make muscle and other tissue, but many proteins also contain phosphate, which can be a problem since it is a large molecule and the dialyser is not very good at removing it. For most people, protein is better taken as lean meat, white fish, or cottage cheese. Vegetarians can maintain their nutrition successfully, but this will need special attention. Extra milk, hard cheese, and eggs should not be used to boost protein intake because they contain a lot of phosphate, but can be taken in moderate amounts. Other protein sources with a very high phosphate are offal (liver, kidneys, etc.), oily fish (salmon, herring, mackerel), and chocolate—which also has a lot of potassium in it (see below).

Salt intake needs to be watched because this can lead to fluid retention and high blood pressure. Particularly salty foods will need to be, in general, avoided, little salt used in cooking, and salt should not be added at the table. Spices starting with the commonly used pepper, but also chives, garlic, basil, mint, and parsley, can be used to give extra flavour to meals.

Some patients have more problems than others with potassium, particularly if they do not have a small amount of kidney function remaining. High potassium foods will need to be avoided as far as possible. These include a number of fruits such as bananas, apricots, all dried fruits, kiwi fruit, and rhubarb. Some vegetables particularly potatoes other than boiled potatoes (boiling takes out the potassium), spinach, and mushrooms, also need to be used with care. Nuts are particularly strong in potassium, as are many breakfast cereals, most wines and most real fruit juices (as opposed to 'fruit' drinks). DON'T use 'salt substitutes' because they are almost all potassium salts, which you must avoid; besides they taste bitter rather than salt, and are not as successful in giving flavour as pepper, etc.

From all this you might think that there is just about nothing you *can* eat! However this is far from the case, and obviously the unit dietician is someone very important for people on haemodialysis for their kidney failure, to guide them in the direction of the many tasty foods which you can eat without restriction. Success with diets requires self-discipline, but at the same time a flexible approach.

What are the complications of being on dialysis?

Successful though long-term dialysis may be, whether in home, in a limited care unit, or in a dialysis centre, it does not return you to completely full health. Rather, it 'freezes' the state of uraemia, with many of the complications of chronic kidney failure (see Chapter 5) still present, plus a few that are peculiar to dialysis. Some of these are trivial; others can be overwhelming. You need to know something about the possible complications of dialysis: fortunately, no-one suffers from all of them at once!

Anaemia and EPO

One main problem is that the majority of even well-dialysed patients remain *anaemic*. This may be a profound anaemia, especially if the kidneys have had to be removed, because this results in a complete lack of the hormone erythropoietin, EPO (see Chapter 1). No patient with one-third of the usual amount of red blood cells can feel anything like 100 per cent, and the amazing fact is how well people can accommodate to anaemia.

In 1986 the first patients on dialysis were treated with biologically engineered EPO, and now perhaps two thirds of patients in the UK and almost all in the USA enjoy the benefit of this treatment. This medicine is given several times a week by injection under the skin, which most people manage without difficulty. Pre-loaded syringes are available to help make the injections easier. A few patients experience pain at the site of the injection, but this is not usually a major problem. If the worst comes to the worst you can have the injection into the vein whilst dialysing.

You might think that it would be best to bring the amount of haemoglobin in the blood back to normal, and this is quite possible using EPO. However, usually the haemoglobin level is adjusted at just below this (at about 11 g/dl, normal 13–15) to avoid complications of EPO treatment. These are a rise in the blood pressure, and clotting of veins or even arteries, especially the vital fistula you need for dialysis.

The other problem with EPO is its high *cost*. Doctors in Britain give EPO to fewer patients than most other countries, largely because of restrictions on the budget available for patients in kidney failure. This cannot be defended.

Itching

Secondly, you may *itch*. This sounds a trivial complaint, but isn't! This is almost certainly a feature of the nerve disease (neuropathy) of the uraemic state, and we have no effective treatment for it; baby oil and sodium bicarbonate in the bath can help, as may low doses of ultraviolet light, but in general little can be done for relief, although some anti-itching tablets help.

High blood pressure

There may be problems with *high blood pressure*, which is intimately connected with the weight and problems with salt intake and limiting fluid intake, since both weight and blood pressure vary rapidly and widely with fluid intake and loss. If too much is gained, then it will have to be removed by increased 'suck' at the next dialysis, which can lead to severe cramp if more than about 2 litres are taken off during an average dialysis. Nowadays, fluid removal is often performed on the same machine before dialysis begins (sequential ultrafiltration) and the patient feels much better using this technique. Medicines may have to be used to lower the blood pressure (for details see Chapter 5), and because the renin level in the blood is high, drugs which inhibit the production of angiotensin (ACE inhibitors, see Chapter 5) are often used.

Bone and joint problems

Bone problems occur in chronic kidney failure (see Chapter 5) and may continue or become worse during dialysis. Usually these don't give rise to anything you will notice, although occasionally, *bone pain* may be a problem, but this is principally found in children. Because dialysis does not adequately control the phosphate in the blood if you are eating a good diet, a medicine must be given to prevent phosphate absorption from food. Usually this takes the form of a calcium salt, often calcium carbonate—common chalk. Sometimes aluminium-containing medicines are used as an alternative or in addition to the calcium carbonate, but in this case the blood level of aluminium needs to be wached carefully, because aluminium is toxic. If bone disease is detected on blood tests, often vitamin D in the form of calcidol (1-alpha) or calitriol (1,25) will be given. Rarely, the parathyroid glands have to be removed from the neck if even vitamin D does not work (see Chapter 5). If you can have a transplant then the parathyroid glands gradually get smaller and the problem subsides, so the decision whether or not to suggest parathyroid removal if you are on dialysis depends to some extent on whether you are likely to get a successful transplant (see Chapter 8).

A joint problem, which is found only in people on long-term dialysis, and which has become apparent as people have spent more than 10 or 15 years on this treatment is *dialysis amyloid*. This is a deposit in the soft tissues and bone round joints, made up of a small protein which is normally got rid of through the kidney but which accumulates in the blood of those on dialysis. Dialysis amyloid never appears before about 7 years' dialysis, but can become a major problem after 10 or 15 years. The main joints affected are the hands, the shoulders, and the spine, in that order of frequency. One of the nerves to the hands (the radial nerve) may be compressed at the wrist when it runs through what is called the carpal tunnel, in the palm of the hand just beyond the crease of the wrist. This may require a small operation to release it. Painful stiff wrists and shoulders are another common problem. At the moment the only solution to this is to try and get a transplant, but it is those patients who are most difficult to transplant and who are on dialysis long term who most often suffer from it.

Psychological problems

More important than all these, however, are the *psychological problems* faced by patients on long-term dialysis. These may amount, at their worst, to an expressed or unexpressed suicide. Different individuals may come to terms with the limitations of their life on regular dialysis in different ways, and in different degrees, according to their individual temperaments, degree of family support, or job. Adolescents and young people find it particularly difficult to accept the ruthless discipline necessary to achieve success on dialysis. Most families report the effects of the stress on one member on dialysis, and some marriages break up under it; equally, others are more securely welded. Depression, sexual impotence in men, and lack of sex urge in females are common complaints, and sexual function is not helped by the hormonal changes of kidney failure and the tiredness of anaemia. Earnings are frequently less than before going on to dialysis, jobs may be difficult to get, money worries pile up, and social life may be limited.

The main stress, however, is the inevitability of having to dialyse three times a week, apparently for ever. Fear of the dialysis going wrong, or more general fears of death, may be particularly evident if there are many technical problems with access or dialysis, especially if it is being done at home. Aggressive behaviour and 'kicking over the traces' with regard to diet and fluids may be signs that help is needed in other directions. The major problem is to get the dialysis procedure into perspective, merely as a means to an end, in spite of the fact that its technical detail and complexity, the new terminology and way of life, may overwhelm patient and family to begin with. You have to learn to dialyse in order to live, not the reverse. Many units have formal or informal patient support groups and/or formal counselling to help you cope and sort out any specific problems.

Lack of mobility for patients on regular dialysis is now less of a problem, and the psychological liberation of being able to enjoy a holiday, at home or abroad, may be great. As mentioned above, many units now have holiday homes or caravans, many units will accept patients from other units for holidays, and the British Kidney Patient Association (see Appendix 2) runs holiday dialysis centres in the UK and abroad. Patients can use portable machines to go away for holidays, and airlines are usually sympathetic in transporting these.

Aluminium poisoning

This is now fortunately of historical interest, but presented a major problem for a while. Now the water used for dialysis contains only tiny amounts of aluminium, whereas in some parts of the country in the past large amounts were added to make the water look clearer. The other source of aluminium is the medicines which contain aluminium given to prevent bone troubles by binding phosphate in the diet. Today all dialysis patients have their aluminium levels checked regularly. The worst form of aluminium poisoning was called *dialysis dementia*. As its name implied, the nervous system was severely affected with loss of mental faculties, beginning with difficulty with speech and incoordination of movement, fits, and then eventually a mute paralysis. Fortunately, no new cases have occurred for many years.

Viruses: hepatitis B and C and HIV (AIDS virus)

Finally, not really a complication of dialysis, but a risk to dialysis patients and dialysis staff, is liver inflammation (hepatitis) from one of several viruses usually called hepatitis viruses A, B, and C. Hepatitis A is the infectious jaundice you can get from contaminated food or water, but hepatitis B and C virus infections are problems in dialysis, since they are usually transmitted by syringes and infected blood. When infected by hepatitis B or C, normal individuals have an acute illness with jaundice, and throw off the virus. Patients on dialysis, or in chronic kidney failure, have a poor immune system just as patients following transplantation do. In all three situations, once the patient has got hepatitis B or C he or she keeps it, becomes a carrier, and their blood is full of the virus for years—usually forever. This makes them highly infectious, since dialysis cannot be performed without blood (the peritoneal fluid in PD is also infected, see Chapter 7). Patients are therefore carefully tested for hepatitis at all stages, and if positive, need to be segregated from other patients to avoid an epidemic. Ironically, the patients remain well (although liver disease may appear after several years) whilst the normal staff members are quite ill if they get it.

Similar considerations hold for those who are HIV positive. They need to have a dialysis machine designated for their use, or to dialyse at home. AIDS itself can cause kidney failure, but the majority of the small number of patients with kidney failure who are HIV positive get it through sexual exposure, or exposure to needles or infected blood.

Summary

Reading the last few pages may make regular dialysis sound like a prolonged torment, which for some it can be; however, for many others it provides a way of life to which they can accommodate for long periods perhaps indefinitely, and which they find preferable to transplantation. Patients have lived on regular haemodialysis for as long as 25 years or even more, and a limit is not yet in sight. Nevertheless, dialysis beyond 10 years needs to be carefully considered in relation to the problems which mount up after that time.

Haemofiltration

This is a technique closely related to haemodialysis, and extends one aspect of that treatment—the removal of water and its salts by filtration under pressure. Using thinner, more permeable membranes in the filter, it is possible to remove many litres of water during a single treatment and replace them with solutions given back into the circuit. These fluids have a composition like dialysate used with the artificial kidney, which resembles that of normal blood plasma water. Unlike dialysis fluids, however, because they are being given into the receiving vein they have to be sterile, like any other intravenous solution. Thus, haemofiltration is much more expensive than haemodialysis or PD, and so has been little used in the UK and the USA; although it is popular in Germany.

It is now the standard treatment, however, for *acute reversible kidney failure*, where costs are less important because the treatment lasts only a few weeks at most. Also, the extra fluid removed allows easier management of these very ill patients, particularly with regard to providing enough food via their veins.

7 Treatments of kidney failure: peritoneal dialysis

This chapter considers the treatment of kidney failure by *peritoneal dialysis* (PD). Because it is a dialysis treatment, it holds you in a state of mild kidney failure, rather than curing it. Peritoneal dialysis has much in common with haemodialysis. The basis of dialysis and uraemia in general have already been discussed; please refer to Chapter 5 about chronic kidney failure, and Chapter 6 on haemodialysis.

Like haemodialysis at home, CAPD is a treatment you give yourself at home, and even at work, during the course of your ordinary day. This has all the advantages and disadvantages you can imagine: the freedom to do it (within limits) at your own convenience, but the responsibility and worries of being responsible for your own treatment and future. Naturally, after training for CAPD you have the backup of the Nephrology team at your unit.

What is the peritoneum?

The peritoneum (Figure 23) is a tough, glistening membrane which covers the guts, liver, stomach, and spleen and which forms a sac into which they protrude or lie free. This permits the bowel to move around as it pushes food through the canal within it. The peritoneal membrane forms an intricate cavity with a large surface area and has a rich blood supply, which allows us to use it for exchange of substances in and out of the body, if fluid is instilled into it, allowed to equilibrate, and then withdrawn again.

History

At the same time as the introduction of *haemodialysis* to the treatment of kidney failure, dialysis using an exchange through the blood vessels in a natural membrane—the peritoneum—rather than through an artificial membrane, was exploited also: *peritoneal dialysis*. It was realized nearly a century ago that dissolved substances would exchange into and out of fluids run into the peritoneal cavity which surrounds the bowel. The problem was—

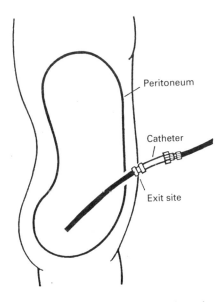

Figure 23 The dialysis catheter is placed into the peritoneal cavity, which contains and surrounds much of your bowel. To make the diagram simple, the loops of bowel within the peritoneal cavity have been left out of the drawing.

and still is—that running even sterile fluid in can lead to infections. Before modern plastics and antibiotics, peritoneal dialysis could make no headway in clinical medicine, although it was tried occasionally starting with the work of Ganter in Germany as long ago as 1923. Between 1955 and 1960 PVC (polyvinylchloride) tubing was introduced into medicine, and with antibiotics available, peritoneal dialysis became rapidly popular as an alternative to haemodialysis for the treatment of acute, reversible kidney failure, especially in children.

However, attempts to use it long-term for irreversible kidney failure were not so successful. Applying the same principles as for acute reversible kidney failure, but on a regular basis, just as had been done in haemodialysis, resulted in an unacceptably high rate of infection within the peritoneum (peritonitis), and patients who were not as well as those who were haemodialysed. In 1969 the introduction of silicone rubber catheters which could be implanted permanently (by Palmer of Vancouver, Canada, and Tenckhoff in Seattle, USA) helped, but the major breakthrough came later, in the middle 1970s: Popovich, an engineer, calculated that one could exploit peritoneal dialysis in a different way, and set out to do this with Jack Moncrief, a nephrologist. Instead of using the technique intermittently, using one or two exchanges of fluid every hour, for two or three days at the most once a week, and then leaving the peritoneum alone, Moncrief and Popovich used *only four exchanges a day—but kept the patient doing this every day of the week*. This continuous slow dialysis with the fluid remaining in the peritoneum for several hours whilst the patient is up and about or sleeping, is usually called CAPD (pronounced 'see A pee dee', or Cap-dee) which stands for the American name, Continuous Ambulatory Peritoneal Dialysis). It is simple to perform, does not necessarily require expensive apparatus, is relatively gentle, and suits many patients very well.

What sort of cannula will be put into my peritoneum? How will it be put in?
Obviously, a first requirement for CAPD is to be able to have long-term access to the peritoneum, to put fluid into and out of the peritoneal cavity. A cannula (catheter) made of silicone rubber about 25 cm (10 inches) long (Plate 19) can be pushed into the cavity in the ward, mounted on a wire to make it stiff. Sterile techniques and local anaesthetic to anaesthetize the skin and peritoneum itself are used, of course, and is done under sedation. Most people rate it as uncomfortable, but not painful. Alternatively the catheter can be put in place under a full general anaesthetic with a minor operation, during which the peritoneal cavity is opened, and the catheter guided in by hand.

In general the simple insertion can be used in those having a first catheter who have not had previous operations in their abdomen, whereas those who have already had a catheter in, or those with previous will probably need the insertion by the small surgical operation with an anaesthetic.

After the cannula has been inserted and strapped into place, fluid can then be run into and out of the abdomen. Usually, however, the catheter will be 'rested' for a couple of days and then used, so that it can heal into place and leaks do not appear when it is first used.

The design of the catheter varies somewhat, but is usually based on one introduced by Tenckhoff of Seattle, and is often referred to by his name. This is a simple tube made of soft silicone rubber with a number of holes near the end which will stay within your abdomen to allow for better fluid drainage, with two cuffs of rough Dacron (R) wool round the catheter near the other end, which are placed just under the skin to promote healing, and to anchor the catheter in place. Further in, there is another similar cuff, placed just before the tube enters the peritoneal cavity. The outer end of the catheter is strapped to the skin and is plugged into a connecting tube which can be changed from time to time; a light dressing covers the exit site of the tube from the abdomen. You will only need to touch the outer end of this connecting tube to change fluid bags (Plate 20).

What fluids will I use to do peritoneal dialysis?

Unlike haemodialysis fluids, peritoneal dialysis fluids *must* be strictly sterile, and are supplied in PVC or polythene bags of 1, 1.5, or 2 litres (2, 3, or 4 pints). The solution is similar to that used for haemodialysis, that is a solution of salts with a controlled low level of acidity—but with one difference: peritoneal dialysis fluid contains a very high concentration of glucose.

This glucose is to allow removal of fluid. There is no way in which negative hydrostatic pressure ('suck') can be applied to the peritoneum, as in haemodialysis, so another feature of diffusion has to be employed. This is, that when the dissolved substances are moving down a concentration gradient, there is a tendency for water to move in the opposite direction, so that equilibrium is reached quickly. Thus, if enough of a bland substance, such as glucose, is put into the peritoneum, there is a tendency for water to enter the peritoneum, independently of the exchange of urea, etc. going on at the same time. If the fluid is then drained out, more water will come out than was put in to begin with. Solutions of various strengths of glucose, usually 15 g/litre (often called a 'weak' or 'normal' bag), 45 g/litre (used occasionally), and 65 g of glucose per litre (a 'strong' or 'heavy' bag), are supplied to achieve the removal of the required amount of fluid, and can be used as required (see below).

What is involved in exchanges of peritoneal dialysis fluid?

To begin with, the two litres of fluid are run into the peritoneum through the cannula using gravity (Figure 24), the empty infusion bag is rolled up and kept in a small pouch in a trouser pocket or under the skirt, and then unrolled at the end of the exchange so that the fluid can be run out into the same bag, again by gravity.

However, today many patients use a so-called 'disconnect' system in which the bag is disconnected from the tube, so that all you have to carry around between exchanges is a short (about 10 cm–4 inches) rubber tube, which is capped off between exchanges.

Either way, the collection bag is weighed to ascertain the volume of fluid that has been extracted (1 litre of solution (2 pints) weighs exactly 1 kilogram (2 pounds)). Usually, because of the glucose in the solution, the volume coming out will generally be greater than that run in—for example 2.4 litres run out, after 2 litres run in. The strength of the glucose in the bag will be chosen to achieve the right fluid loss over a day, and you must weigh yourself

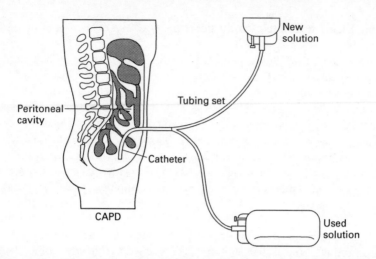

Figure 24 Exchanges using the basic peritoneal dialysis circuit. The full length of the tubing is not shown—normally the bags of fluid (each containing 1.5-2.0 litres or 3-4 pints) are hung high to run the fluid in under gravity. After the dwell in the peritoneum—overnight or after 4 hours or so during the day—then the bag is placed on a clean surface on the floor the clips on the exit tubing opened, and the fluid runs out, again under gravity. Then the bag is disconnected, and another fresh bag of fluid hung up and run in. After this the bag may be rolled up and kept in a pocket or under a skirt. In 'disconnect' systems, the bag is removed from the catheter, and a new connection made to run in the next bag. As a result, there is always about 2 litres of fluid (4 pints) inside the abdomen, which is never completely empty.

daily to see that has been achieved: in the short term, changes in weight are dependent entirely on changes in body fluids. Blood pressure checks are also necessary because this goes up and down with too much or too little fluid in the body.

Because of the danger of infection within the peritoneum (peritonitis, see below), the disconnection and connection need to be done in a sterile fashion. To help this, usually the connector at the end of the tube is kept covered with antiseptic, and the tube is flushed through with antiseptic before fluid is run in. Thus the system is often referred to as 'flush before fill', and has cut down the amount of peritonitis considerably.

How often do I need to do exchanges?

Most patients do four exchanges each day: in the morning before the working day, another at midday, another about 6 p.m., and another before going to bed.

Thus, only one bag is needed at work, at the lunch-break; some patients need only three exchanges each day. For the exchange, you need only a reasonably clean surface, but free from dust and dry. Most homes and workplaces have somewhere an exchange can be done. The time taken to drain the fluid out, disconnect, reconnect, and run in another bag varies somewhat, but usually takes an hour or less including set-up time.

It is common to need three 15 g/l 'normal' strength glucose bags, and one 'strong' 65 g/l glucose bag, which is usually left in overnight. However this routine may be varied according to need; if weight is being gained and you are becoming swollen, it may be necessary to use more strong (70 g/l) bags for a while. The unit staff will work it out with you at the beginning, and revise from time to time, what target weight (often referred to as 'dry' weight) you need to keep to.

Do I need to come to hospital?

To begin with you will need to come to the hospital or CAPD training centre to learn how to do the exchanges and to care for your catheter. This training period varies, but is usually 7–10 days. After that, once a month or two months, you will need to come up to the unit to have your external connector changed by one of the unit staff. Otherwise the catheter and its junction with the connector is left alone, although the dressing (if one is used) over it is changed. These meticulous details are necessary because of the risk of peritonitis, which is the most important complication of CAPD. It is possible to bathe and to swim. However the exit site remains perhaps the most vulnerable point in the CAPD system.

How do I get supplies for CAPD at home?

The unit responsible for your treatment will order the necessary bags, connection sets and fluids, etc., to be delivered to your home. When you are established on treatment you will be able to do this yourself. Obviously it helps to have some in reserve in case the delivery from the manufacturer is late. Space will be needed to store the bags, etc., which take up a fair bit of room, as you are using 57 litres (112 pints) a week of fluid; a month's supply takes up as much room as 200 pint bottles of milk!

Who can have CAPD?

Very few people cannot do CAPD. It works well in tiny infants and old people as well as older children and adults. Those who have had operations or problems with their peritoneum are often not able to use it for CAPD. Some degree of dexterity is required, and of course ordinarily you need reasonable eyesight. Thus there are considerable extra difficulties for people with shaky hands or arthritis, or with poor eyesight that cannot be corrected (for example by spectacles or having a cataract removed). However gadgets exist to help putting the tubes together for connection and disconnection, so that even completely blind people (for example as a result of diabetes) can do CAPD successfully. CAPD requires no apparatus, allows you great mobility; but takes up about 4 hours each day, during which you will need to sit, for example in a chair.

It is obvious that CAPD is much simpler to do than haemodialysis, can be done at home as a routine, and frees you from attendance at hospital dialysis unit three times a week. It is much gentler than haemodialysis and therefore suits patients with poor heart function, which is the case with many elderly patients, especially those with poor heart function, which is the case with many elderly patients, especially those with widespread blood vessel disease. However it is not so suitable for big, muscular people, being best for smaller individuals, who produce less of the poisonous substances that need to be dialysed off. Whilst it is usually possible to carry on with haemodialysis for many years, only about half of patients started on CAPD are able to continue the treatment for more than five years. Nevertheless some patients have gone beyond 10 years on CAPD without a break. Because CAPD has only been in widespread use for about 12-14 years, we do not know in the very long term how well the technique will serve.

Holidays are much easier to take with CAPD than with haemodialysis, since all that need be arranged is the transport or delivery of the CAPD bags to the hotel, or even campsite. One *can* do CAPD almost anywhere, even in a train or on a beach, although you need to be even more careful about your technique under these circumstances. Fluid restriction is usually less strict than on haemodialysis but is still important—most patients will need to drink no more than 1-1.5 litres (2-3 pints) a day. Also for reasons which are not clear, anaemia is less severe on CAPD than on haemodialysis and fewer patients on CAPD need treatment with EPO.

Automated (machine) peritoneal dialysis (APD, CCPD)

An alternative way of doing peritoneal dialysis is to use a machine (a PD cycler) which cycles the fluid in and out of the peritoneum automatically (Plate 21). This is an advantage for patients who cannot make exchanges during the day, or who cannot manage to learn the technique of CAPD at all. APD is usually done each night whilst you are asleep for 8–10 hours, and has the advantage of not requiring exchanges during the day. These machines are much smaller and much simpler to run than a haemodialysis monitor, but must be set up with enough bags of fluid (which are much larger than those used for the individual exchanges of CAPD) before use. Peritonitis rates are generally lower than with CAPD (see below) and the main disadvantage of this technique is one of cost, which is very high compared with even haemodialysis in the hospital unit. Thus it has not much been used in the UK, but is becoming increasingly popular worldwide.

What complications might I get during CAPD?

Some general complications of CAPD are those which depend upon the continued presence of higher levels of potentially toxic substances in the blood than in health. These have been discussed in Chapter 5, and in Chapter 6 on haemodialysis. They include the risk of bone and joint problems, and as in people on haemodialysis treatment, it may be necessary to take medicines to limit the level of phosphate in the blood to prevent bone problems, and if this fails vitamin D or even removal of the parathyroid glands in the neck may be necessary (see Chapters 5 and 6). In addition, the psychological problems of adapting to a life on dialysis are much the same as for haemodialysis, although of course there is no need to needle veins, which is a big advantage. The difference in CAPD is the attitude to the tube hanging from the abdomen, which some people have no problems with, but others find repugnant.

However there are some additional problems also which relate directly to the technique of CAPD. The most important of these is peritonitis.

Peritonitis

This is the main problem with CAPD. Germs get into the peritoneum down the track of the catheter, from the skin, and in some older people with chronic inflammation of the large bowel (diverticulitis) through the bowel wall. Since peritonitis is the major short-term limitation on CAPD, much effort has been put into trying to find out why it happens. Sometimes it is the fault of sloppy technique, but often it seems to occur 'out of the blue'. Recently, many doctors have come to accept that inevitably the peritoneum will be contaminated with germs from time to time—perhaps at low level *all* the time, and rather than trying to prevent this fruitlessly, they have turned their attention to making sure that any germs present are killed. This is done by the 'flush before fill' systems described above, or by surrounding the connection with a box which irradiates it with ultraviolet (UV) light.

How will I know if I have peritonitis, and how will it be treated?   If you have peritonitis, you will notice several things. First, the fluid draining out of your abdomen, instead of being a clear straw colour, becomes cloudy. Second, you may experience a variable amount of pain in your abdomen, especially if there is any pressure on it. Finally, you may feel generally unwell, with a mounting fever, loss of appetite, and all the symptoms of severe infection. Because the peritoneum is so large, the organisms (germs) responsible can get into the bloodstream very easily. Treatment is with antibiotics, usually injected directly into the bags, as well as by mouth or by injection.

Usually peritonitis will require a visit to the unit, but most often can be cared for at home. However if the germs get into the bloodstream in large numbers you could be ill enough to need to be in hospital for a few days. Treatment will usually last for 7–10 days, and in the great majority of cases, the infection clears up.

However, if there is not rapid resolution of your symptoms, or an unusual organism is found (for example the yeast which causes thrush, called candida) then it may be necessary to remove the catheter, and use haemodialysis for a time. For this reason, if you are going to be on CAPD for more than a short while, you will need a fistula in your arm as back-up should in case you need haemodialysis at any time (see Chapter 6 about fistulae for haemodialysis). Otherwise, the haemodialysis would have to be done temporarily via a neck line, or subclavian line (see Chapter 6).

At the moment, many patients can go long periods without any problems from peritonitis, but a proportion (perhaps a quarter) have to abandon the technique within two years because of recurrent attacks.

Exit site infections

Normally the exit site—the hole through which the catheter emerges—is clean and dry, but it may become wet, scabby, and discharge clear fluid or even pus. This can be a tremendous nuisance, and of course makes an attack of peritonitis more likely. It is treated with antibiotics and dressings. Occasionally an exit site infection is so persistent that the site of the cannula may have to be changed.

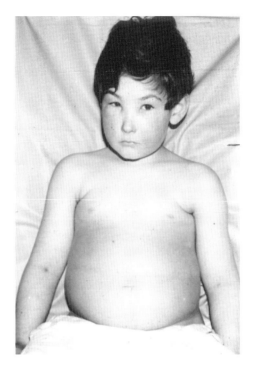

Plate 1 The swelling of kidney disease—the nephrotic syndrome. Puffiness around the eyes is particularly characteristic of kidney disease. Fortunately, in his case the loss of protein was from a reversible problem in the filters (glomeruli) and although he had several attacks of swelling he did not develop kidney failure.

Plate 2 A dipstick used to find abnormal substances in the urine. The lower strip has been dipped in the urine and the right had test square, dark blue in the original, (arrow) which indicates that this urine contains an abnormally large amount of blood. Protein glucose, bile, and acidity can be registered on the other test squares along the strip.

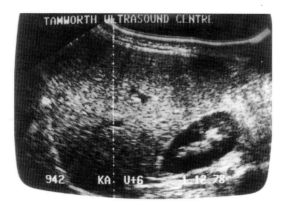

Plate 3 An ultrasound picture of the kidney (K). The ultrasound beam is 'swept' across the organ to be examined, and the echoes of the objects within the beam registered. The kidney substance is seen as the dark, echo-free area, and inner part of the kidney around the calyces as the white area within the kidney. This gives a 'slice' across the kidney, which can be compared with the lower half of Figure 4.

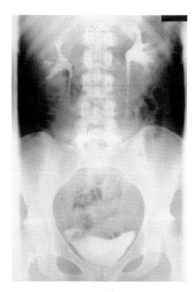

Plate 4 A normal intravenous urogram (IVU), taken 20 minutes after the injection of contrast into a vein in the arm. The collecting system of the kidney, the pelvis (p), the ureters draining the urine (u) to the bladder (b) can all seen in white, since the contrast being excreted in the urine is opaque to X-rays. The outline of the bones can be seen also, including the ribs at the top, and the pelvis at the bottom of the picture. Compare with Figure 1.

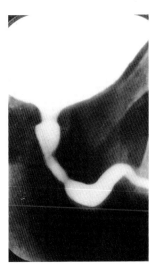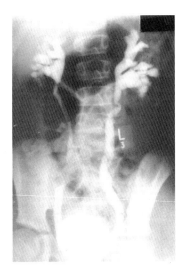

Plate 5 A micturating cysto-urethogram (MCU). The radio-opaque contrast placed into the bladder through a catheter passed in through the urethra is seen (left) outlining the urethra in a 15 year old boy with a congenital obstruction to the upper third of his urethra (arrowed), and kidney failure. The contrast flows backwards (reflux) up from the bladder into the ureters to outline the whole urinary tract, almost like the picture on the IVU (Plate 4) but in this case the kidney outline is abnormal. In a normal individual, only the bladder would be outlined and the rest of the urinary tract would not be seen.

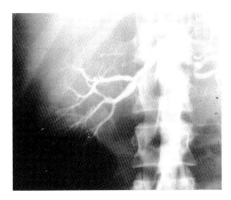

Plate 6 An arteriogram of the blood supply to the kidney. The white area shows the main artery of the body, the aorta (A), from which the arteries to the kidneys branch directly. There is a narrowing of the artery to the kidney. Behind the aorta, the vertebrae of the spine can be seen, and the ribs at top left.

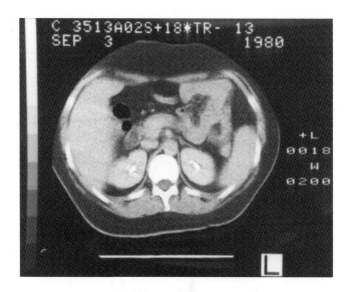

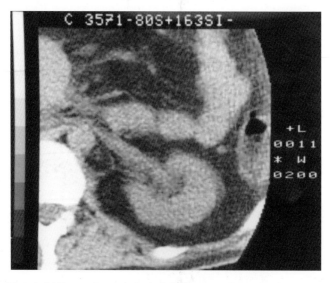

Plate 7 (Top) A CAT scan showing the kidneys (K) on either side of the spine (S). This shows a whole 'slice' through the body at the level of the kidneys: the skin, muscles, spleen (on the left in front of the kidney), and the intestines can be seen, as varying densities of the X-ray picture. (Bottom) A more detailed view of the kidney is seen. The collecting system (pelvis and ureter) can be seen within the kidney substance.

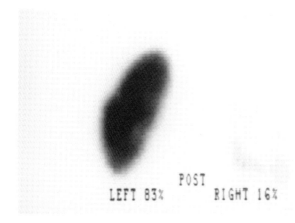

POST

LEFT 83%   RIGHT 16%

Plate 8 A particular radioactive compound, called DMSA, has been injected when accumulates in the kidney. By counting all the radioactivity within the area of the kidney the function of each kidney can be estimated, as well as obtaining an outline of the kidney to look for scars or other abnormalities. In this case the right kidney is extremely small, and has very poor function.

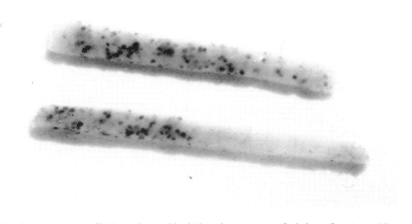

Plate 9 A tiny piece of kidney obtained by kidney biopsy, magnified about five times. The glomerular filters are diseased and therefore more visible than usual. They can be seen as the dark dots in the biopsy cores. The upper piece of the biopsy contains only cortex, but in the lower core the junction of the cortex (C) and the medulla (M) can be seen. The biopsy is fixed, thin slices taken and stained with various reagents to examine the structure of the filters (glomeruli) and the tubules under the microscope.

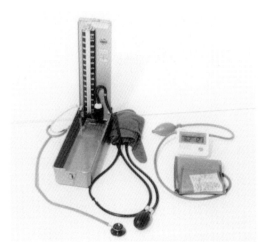

Plate 10 Two blood pressure machines. On the left is the classical mercury sphygomanometer. The pressure in the cuff around the arm is measured directly by the height of a column of mercury, and the sounds are listened to over an artery, during the gentle deflation of the pressure within the cuff. On the right is an automatic machine, which reads the blood pressure out digitally after sensing the vibrations from the blood vessel during deflation of the cuff. In some models the cuff is automatically inflated and deflated.

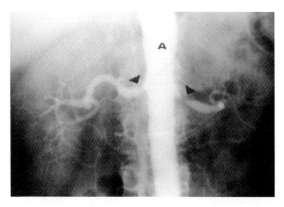

Plate 11 Blockage of both renal arteries by degeneration (atheroma) of the blood vessels. The main artery from the heart the aorta (A) and the arteries to the kidneys on either side have been rendered visible on X-ray by doing an aortogram, which involves injecting a dye, which shows as white in the picture (see Plate 6). Both the renal arteries supplying the kidneys are narrowed (arrowheads). The narrowings are progressive and eventually cut off the blood supply to the kidneys completely.

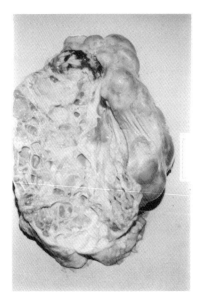

Plate 12 A polycystic kidney. It is enormous—about 25 cm (8–10 inches) long compared with the normal 10–12 cm (4–41/2 inches). The whole surface and substance of the kidney is occupied with multiple cysts most of which contain clear fluid, but in some is turbid or contains blood.

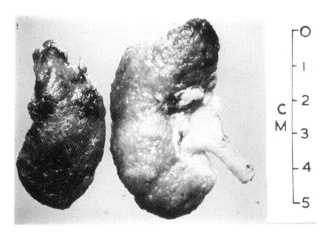

Plate 13 The tiny, coarsely scarred kidneys of someone with severe progressive scarring as a result of reflux of urine and high blood pressure. Normal kidneys, for comparison (Chapter 1) are 10–12 cm long.

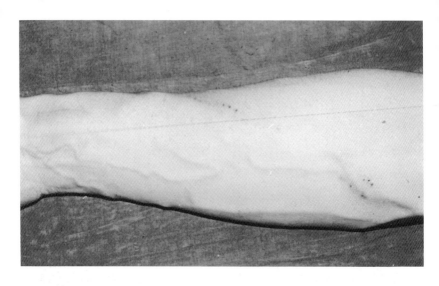

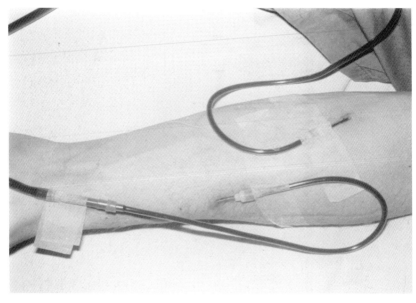

Plate 14 An arteriovenous fistula (top photograph) with needles inserted for dialysis (bottom).

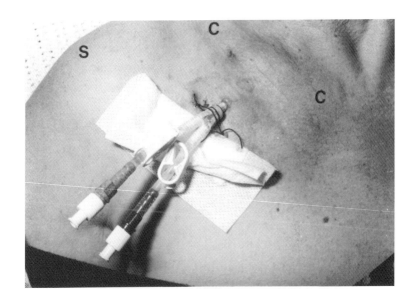

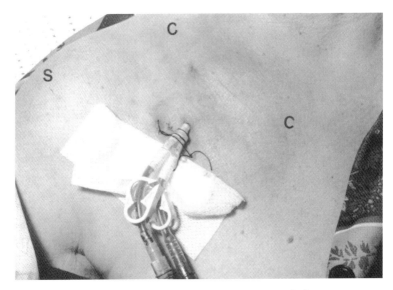

Plate 15 A subclavian catheter in place (top) and the two channels forming it connected up for dialysis (bottom).

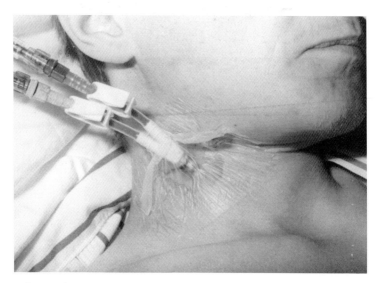

Plate 16 A 'neck line' in the internal jugular vein connected to two lines for haemodialysis.

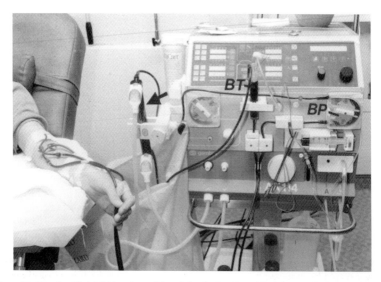

Plate 17 The 'artificial kidney' machine. The 'kidney' itself is the small dialyzer (arrow) whilst the machine makes fluid for dialysis, pumps blood through a blood pump (BP) and prevents air bubbles re-entering the blood stream in a bubble trap (BT) in the blood line.

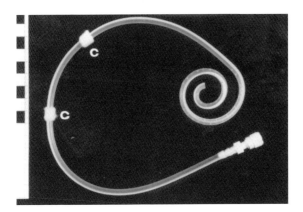

Plate 18 A peritoneal dialysis catheter, made from silicone rubber. The two cuffs of wooly Dacron (C) are placed beneath the skin but outside the peritoneum to help anchor the catheter firmly in place. The curled portion of the catheter is inside the peritoneal cavity, and has a number of tiny holes to make drainage of fluid easier. At the other end is the connector for making the connection to the line from the bags of fluid.

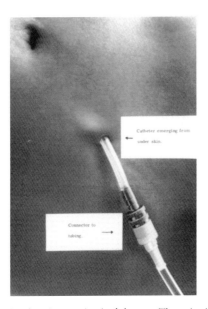

Plate 19 The catheter in place in a patient's abdomen. The exit site where the catheter emerges should be clean and free of debris and dry. The catheter itself is joined through a titanium connector to an intermediate tube which is changed at the hospital every two months or so (bottom left) and this connects with the disposable parts of the drainage circuit. This catheter has a metal connector; plastic is more usual today.

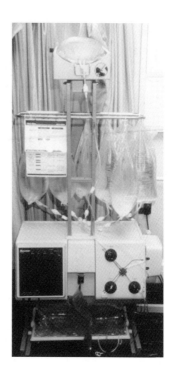

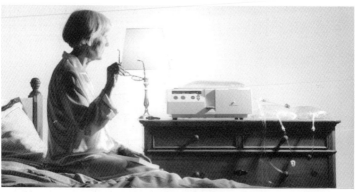

Plate 20 (Top) A machine for doing APD—Automated PD, also called CCPD (continuous cycling PD). This one is similar in size to a haemodialysis machine, and carries the large bags of peritoneal dialysis fluid. (Bottom) The much smaller 'HomeChoice' system (Baxter Healthcare). It weighs 11 kg (22 lbs) and so is just portable. In both cases, the dialysis is usually done overnight to allow greater freedom, and the machine does all the switching and pumping of fluid necessary to perform the dialysis, rather than doing it by hand as in conventional PD.

Hernias

If you already have a hernia, it will need to be repaired before you start CAPD. CAPD also brings on hernias because of the weight of fluid inside the abdomen, and especially older patients may develop hernias which need attention. Obviously an operation will be required to repair the hernia and the CAPD will have to be stopped temporarily, and you will need haemodialysis in the meantime.

Back pain

Many patients have mild back pain but in a few people it is a severe problem and may lead to CAPD being abandoned. This is not common however.

Blood vessel disease

The continuous infusion of glucose from the bags into the patients alters the blood fats, and whether this will prove to be a factor increasing blood vessel diseases (e.g. myocardial infarcts) remains to be seen.

What medicines will I need to take whilst on CAPD?

In general the only medicines that will be needed will be:

(i)   *Iron*, because it is absorbed poorly if you are uraemic.

(ii)   *Vitamins*, because some of them are dialysed out in the PD fluid. However, if you are eating a well-balanced diet containing enough vitamins these may not be necessary.

(iii) *Phosphate binders*. Medicines to take phosphate out of your blood (*phosphate binders*), such as calcium carbonate (chalk) or aluminium hydroxide, will usually be necessary since if you eat enough protein to make up for the losses of protein from your CAPD fluid, then you will at the same time be taking in phosphate.

(iv)   If your bones are giving problems (see Chapter 5) then it may be necessary to take a small dose of a *vitamin D* preparation such as calcitriol or 1-alpha to protect your bones, but unfortunately this often leads to the calcium level in the blood going too high.

(v)   If you have high blood pressure despite CAPD—which is quite common—then you may need tablets to help lower your blood pressure. Details of the various medicines used for this are given in Chapter 4.

(vi)   If your haemoglobin remains low despite adequate dialysis, you may need EPO injections.

(vii) Constipation is a common problem in patients doing CAPD, and if severe interferes with your exchanges. Thus you may need to take *laxatives*. Don't buy these yourself from the chemists because some of these are unsuitable for someone like you without kidneys; ask the unit staff about this.

(viii) Obviously also, diabetics will need to continue their insulin injections, or tablets, to control their diabetes. Some anti-diabetic tablets are unsuitable for people in kidney failure, and may have to be changed to ones which are got rid of by the liver rather than the kidneys.

The effect of the glucose going into the peritoneum on the diabetes is surprisingly small.

One can give the insulin with the sugar, into each bag before it is run in, but although this has advantages, this is tedious and injecting the bag every time carries an extra risk of infection.

Similarly, for some other diseases which cause kidney failure, the treatment for these may have to be continued whilst on CAPD.

Is diet important on CAPD?

As in haemodialysis (see Chapter 6) diet is *extremely* important for patients on CAPD, especially as in CAPD to some extent you have to do a balancing act: for example, between a lot of protein to make good the losses from the CAPD fluid, which gives you more phosphate than you can handle; or vegetables and fruit to give you necessary vitamins, which can raise the level of potassium in your blood too high.

Because you are losing a lot of protein in the CAPD fluid—about the equivalent of the whites of four or five eggs a day—you need to make sure you have a good protein intake. This is better taken as lean meat, white fish, or cottage cheese. Extra milk, hard cheese, and eggs should not be used to boost protein intake because they contain a lot of phosphate, but can be taken in moderate amounts. Other protein sources with a very high phosphate level are offal (liver, kidneys, etc.), oily fish (salmon, herring, mackerel) and chocolate—which also has a lot of potassium in it (see below). There are major problems for vegetarians in doing CAPD to keep up with the protein losses, but it is worth a trial to see if the concentration of albumin the blood can be maintained successfully. Salt intake also needs to be watched (see Chapter 6) and some patients have more problems than others with potassium.

Because you are getting on average about 1500 kCalories from the glucose in the fluid every day, you will need to watch how much carbohydrate (sugar and starch) and fat is in your diet. Many patients on CAPD put on an alarming amount of fat very quickly, and become overweight.

How much will being on CAPD alter my lifestyle?

This very much depends upon you—particularly upon the attitude you take to being a patient in kidney failure on treatment. You should not regard yourself as an invalid, but someone who has to take a rather tedious treatment in order to lead as normal a life as possible. As with haemodialysis, you must dialyse to live, not live to dialyse. Naturally, some people find achieving this more difficult than others. There is no reason why all but the heaviest physical jobs should not be continued or restarted. Holidays are relatively easy compared with haemodialysis, if you give your unit notice to get the bags, etc. delivered to your holiday address.

Your catheter should not interfere with sexual activity. But as discussed in relation to haemodialysis in Chapter 6, the many important changes that take place in your life and the extra worries about the future may affect how you feel about sex. For example, some people feel badly their apparent loss of independence as an individual, or as a breadwinner. Not all patients on dialysis are as well as we or they would like, and poor nutrition, anaemia, and the hormonal changes of uraemia which are not always reversed by dialysis may all affect sexual drive or performance. In addition, some of the drugs used to treat high blood pressure may have an adverse effect (see Chapter 4). Finally some people find that being on dialysis, and particularly the catheter in their abdomen, makes them less attractive, or that they may damage it by sexual activity. These fears need to be brought out into the open and discussed with the Nephrology team, especially the unit counsellor.

Summary

Peritoneal dialysis now forms an important part of our treatment of renal failure, and more than half of the patients in the UK on dialysis use it. For some patients it provides a very acceptable long-term solution, and for others a quick way of starting and continuing dialysis while they wait for a transplanted kidney (see Chapter 8). However, it still has a higher rate of technical failure in the long term than haemodialysis, and is best suited to smaller patients who still have a tiny function left in their kidneys and still pass some urine. Nevertheless, it provides a useful form of treatment for large numbers of patients worldwide.

8 *Kidney transplantation*

A man of my kidney!
Shakespeare: *The Merry Wives of Windsor*, 111, v, 117.

By the end of 1993, about 140 000 patients owed their lives to kidney transplants world-wide, including 64 000 in Europe (12 000 in the UK) and 50 000 in the USA. Every year, 11 000 transplants are done in Europe and almost 10 000 in the USA, of which some 3200 are from living related donors. In addition an unknown number of living donor transplants are done in developing countries—probably another 5000. Despite all the problems which remain unsolved, a successful renal transplant is the most satisfactory treatment for end-stage kidney failure from the medical, psychological, social, and economic points of view. It is now an established form of medical treatment for what was formerly an inevitably fatal condition. This chapter gives you the background to having a kidney transplant, and tells you what you may expect from being considered as a recipient of such a graft, through to the long-term outcomes.

Why can't we just transplant from anyone to anyone?

This is a simple, obvious, and important question, but unfortunately has a complicated answer. In brief, because we are capable of recognizing our own cells as 'self' and attacking anything else and destroying it. This is because for millions of years living organisms have carved out their niche amongst a multitude of others; most organisms form some part of the food chain or another (in this respect we are fortunate!). In particular, multicellular organisms like man have had to make their way in the midst of a universe crowded with micro-organisms: virsuses, bacteria, yeasts, parasites—all eager to multiply within and on us.

To fend off these unwelcome boarders, we have had to evolve a series of mechanisms to defend ourselves. This involves two processes: first the identification of the 'enemy' organism, and second its destruction. To this end, a machinery of *self-identification* has been developed, which we still understand only imperfectly. All the time, cells roam the body 'examining' the surfaces of

Box 4   A little history

Technical problems of transferring organs from one individual to another and connecting them up were solved early in this century. However, simply being able to sew the blood vessels together did not make for successful organ transplantation, and the few attempts at transplanting organs during the 1920s and 1930s all resulted in early failure. During and after World War II, work by Sir Peter Medawar and others showed clearly that the process of rejection of skin grafts was an immunological one which involved information about the 'foreignness' of the graft which was carried by white blood cells of the lymphocyte series; and that the rejection of these grafts again principally involved cells, rather than antibodies free in the circulation.

This led to attempts to blunt or abolish both the recognition or the destruction of the graft; this work is still in progress. The first attempts to perform renal transplantation in animals followed in the early 1950s in Great Britain and the USA, and occasional desperate attempts were made to transplant human kidneys. All failed after days, weeks, or at most months. In Boston, doctors reasoned that, since identical twins were incapable of rejecting skin (this is still one of the tests for confirming that twins are identical), then a kidney transplant should not be rejected either. Late in 1954, the first successful long-term human kidney transplant was undertaken, between identical twins. A number of other twins were transplanted, but, of course, this could benefit only a tiny number of individuals; but by 1959 the technique was extended to transplantation between brothers and sisters who were not twins, in Paris as well. To modify the rejection process, the doctors treated the recipients with whole-body gamma irradiation at a level just below that which would kill them, in an attempt to blunt the rejection process. Two patients given such transplants in 1959 still survived with their grafts in the early 1990s.

Then in 1962, after an exhaustive series of tests on a variety of drugs, the new drug azathioprine (Imuran) was shown by Sir Roy Calne to be a most effective and relatively safe immunosuppressive agent in dogs, especially in combination with prednisone. In fact, this combination was so successful that there was little investigation of alternatives in man until recently. From 1962 to 1965, a large number of living donor transplants were done, notably by Tom Starzl in Colorado in the United States, and it was learned that the ABO blood group system must be respected in organ transplantation. That is, donors and recipients of kidneys had to be blood group compatible. Meanwhile, cautious experiments went ahead to attempt the use of kidneys from individuals who had just died—cadaver donor transplantation. By 1965 it was obvious that these could be made to work in some patients, and renal transplantation units opened all over the world.

The overall results, however, were disappointing. Less than half the cadaver transplants worked, many recipients died, and many of those surviving were damaged by the high doses of prednisone given. Advances in knowledge of the system responsible for recognition of 'foreign-ness' (tissue types, the HLA system) did not seem to lead to any improvement in results, even when the recipient and the donor were 'well' matched; live donor transplantation showed 25–30 per cent better survival at 2–5 years than cadaver transplants, and tissue matching did make a considerable difference in these results with family donors. From 1970 to about 1980 cadaver transplantation, although very active in terms of increasing numbers, stagnated in terms of successful results.

Since then we have moved into a period of progress. Some of this has resulted simply from doing the same things better and promptly. Better, more fresh donor kidneys have become available, because of changed laws, but principally because of greater public awareness and generosity. Transplant units have become more experienced in both transplantation and the management of immunosuppressive drugs, blood transfusion may have had an effect (see below), and now we begin to understand why 'old style' tissue matching did not work.

Next, much improved immunosuppressive agents, particularly cyclosporine (Cyclosporin A, Sandimmun, Neoral) have been introduced. The effect of all this has been that 9 out of 10 of cadaver donor grafts are working at the end of the first year, and three quarters, rather than only half, are still working after 5 years. Nevertheless, there is still plenty of room for improvement, especially in the longer term, when donors from living relatives still do much better than cadaver grafts.

---

any cells they encounter to see whether they 'pass' as self or not. Recognition of 'not-self' usually results in the launching of a series of mechanisms which attack the cell (or cells) identified as foreign, and destroy it. This system may also be used to weed out 'rogue' cells within the body which become different from others, i.e. step outside the body's organization and may begin what we recognize finally as cancerous growths.

If we wish to transplant from one individual to another without restraint, we have to

1) prevent recognition of the foreignness, or

2) blunt the attack reaction.

At the moment, clinical transplantation mostly relies on *blunting the attack reaction* to the foreign organ, using non-specific drugs. What I have just written implies that we should blunt the attack *specifically*—that is, direct it against only the transplanted organ. This is at the moment impossible. The inevitable result of our efforts using drugs to blunt the *whole* immune reaction, to prevent its attack on the grafted kidney, lays the patient open to all the invaders the reaction was designed to repel. Little wonder then, that even today the commonest cause of the rare deaths in transplant recipients is still infection. They may also be more liable than normal to develop tumorous growths, benign or malignant.

Box 5   Tissue typing and transplant antibodies

Tissue typing

Most people are familiar with the fact that red blood cells have a specific type, or group: A, B, AB, or neither A nor B, called O. In fact, for successful transplantation the blood group must be compatible with that of the recipient; Os can only have an O kidney, whilst AB can have any type. As can have A or O, and those with blood group B, similarly B or O.

First in mice and then in humans, it was realized by the mid-1960s that one particular part of the DNA which makes up our chromosomes (Chapter 4) (it is found on chromosome number 6), carried information which determines the production of a series of 'recognition' or 'self' proteins on the surfaces of cells. Since all cells in the body have the same DNA, being descended from a single cell after fertilization, these proteins are present on *all* cells of the body (except the red cells of the blood) to a greater or lesser extent. In practice, the *white* cells of the blood are often used for tissue typing, that is, testing to see which cell surface markers are present in any individual because they are easy to get and easy to work with. Thus, the system came to be called HLA, from Human Leucocyte (white cell) Antigen.

The part of the DNA which codes for these proteins of the HLA system is called the MHC, or major histocompatibility (tissue matching) complex. This complex has a number of sub-divisions, called *sub-loci*, and designated A, B, C, DR, DQ, et. At *each* of these any individual has two units of DNA, one of which has come from the father, and one from the mother. A typical tissue type report will read something like this: HLA: A2, A9; B12, B18; DR3, DR7 (the C locus does not seem to be important in transplantation). But do *all* of them matter? It is now clear that the tissue-typing of the A and B sub-loci, which were performed in the 1960s and early 1970s, was looking at the wrong end of the complex. The A sub-locus seem to matter rather little, the B rather more, but both seem to be of less importance compared with the DR and its closely related systems such as DQ. Unfortunately, unlike blood groups, there are many many different types at each of the four loci of the HLA complex, so that it is very unlikely to find a perfect 6-antigen match in the general population.

However, we are back in a mood of optimism that tissue type matching between donor and recipient *can* make an impact on clinical transplantation: a cadaver transplant with a 'full house' match of all six A, B, and DR antigens between the donor and the recipient survives 15% better at 5 years than one with only one match, or no match at all. The difference seems to get bigger with time, so that really long term survivals are much more likely with a good match.

Transplantation antibodies

There is another group of patients for whom tissue type matching (even of the A and B loci) is absolutely *vital*. These are patients who have developed a large number of circulating antibodies directed against these very same HLA antigens A and B. These antibodies may be the result of previous pregnancy in women, since half any baby's tissue type is necessarily the same as the father's, and the baby can immunize the mother through sharing a circulation.

Unfortunately, it can also result from previous transfusion. But the largest group awaiting a graft who have antibodies have acquired them from a previous failed transplant. The results of these antibodies are usually expressed as the percentage of the normal population against whom antibodies have formed, since this determines how likely it is to find a compatible cadaver donor.

This is usually called the *panel reactivity*, and is expressed from 0 to 100%. Thus if you have 75% panel reactivity, it means that your blood serum contains antibodies which are capable of killing the cells from 75% of a normal population group. Obviously the higher the figure, the more difficult it will be to get a cadaver donor kidney which suits you. It is also necessary to check the particular HLA antigen(s) against which the antibodies are directed, so that one can avoid putting in a kidney which bears these particular antigens. Normally for a second kidney, one would try and avoid all the antigens present on the first kidney which were different from the recipients. Hence the long wait for exactly the right kidney. Large national or international pools of kidneys help to achieve this, and some patients even have kidneys from abroad if one cannot be found in their own country.

Fortunately, these antibodies may gradually fade away, and make finding a suitable donor easier, but equally some patients have so many persistent antibodies that with current techniques they are almost untransplantable, and must wait on regular dialysis treatment until some new advance permits to attack their problem again (see Chapter 11). At the moment different ways of getting rid of these antibodies are being tried, but none are effective in every case, although some successes have been achieved.

The other point is that if transplantation is done despite these antibodies, a very severe rapid form of rejection may occur, called *hyperacute rejection*. This normally happens within hours or days of transplantation, but occasionally happens later—up to a week or two—if the cells making the antibodies take time to get going, and no antibodies are actually present in the circulation when the transplant is done, but the cells with the potential to make them are already present from previous sensitization.

What can we do under the heading of *preventing recognition of foreignness*? At the moment, in terms of clinical transplantation, not much, although we can achieve this in animals using various strategies. But that little has perhaps been enough to allow us to use gentler suppression of immune responses and succeed in keeping the graft in place as well as the patient safe from infection. The first thing we could do would be to find for each individual recipient, amongst all the donors, an 'identical twin' in terms of tissue matching. This is far from easy to do. Even with national organizations for sharing kidneys it is impossible to match exactly more than one patient in 6 for even the main tissue (HLA) types we know about—although this does improve results a significant amount, and explains why most people have to wait for the right cadaver kidney to come up. Now we know that the tissue typing situation is even more complicated than we thought, and this is discussed in Box 5.

The other alternative would be to present the foreign kidney in such a way that the recipient cells accepted it as 'self'. This is an area into which a huge amount of effort has been put.

Put simply, when confronted with a new, recognizable piece of cell surface (an antigen, see below) the body has two choices: accept or reject. Many of the problems lie in our ignorance of how this system operates, and what switch determines which response is evoked. It is clear that anything present before birth (and in mice and rats until just after birth) will be accepted thereafter as 'self'.

Where can we get kidneys from?

There are basically four sources of kidneys:

(1) related individuals who wish to give a kidney (related living donors);

(2) unrelated individuals who wish to give a kidney (unrelated living donors);

(3) unrelated individuals who have just died (cadaver donors);

(4) animal kidneys (xenografted kidneys, from the Greek xen- meaning foreign, stranger).

What about living donor transplantation?

For most purposes in developed countries, this implies *related* living donor transplantation. Because of the considerations of tissue typing (see Box 5), the only relatives close enough to be worth considering strongly (i.e. likely to share a major proportion of their tissue type) are father, mother, brother, sister, daughter, son, although with the use of cyclosporine this has changed. Uncles, aunts, or grandparents are only likely to share one in four of the tissue types, which is little better than could be obtained by matching a cadaver graft, but on occasions have been worth considering. Similar considerations come up when someone caring, but unrelated would like to give a kidney.

Of course, someone must *want* to give a kidney. One might think that always, everyone possible in a family would want to give a kidney, and the surgeons would be only too happy to put it into the recipient. In fact, it's not nearly so simple!

The problems are less for parents of affected children, but even here loyalties may be divided between the desire to provide for one child, whilst inevitably depriving the other children of one parent for a period. This is not a trivial consideration, since the suggestion of transplantation may come after a prolonged illness for the affected child, during which the other children have been (or feel themselves to be) deprived of their full share of parental love. Also, the parents must face up to the possibility that, despite their sacrifice, the kidney may not function usefully, and all will have been in vain. Finally, there may be conflict between the parents as to who should give a kidney, everything else being equal; unspoken and overt marital conflicts may surface at this point.

With brothers and sisters the problem is sometimes obvious. Divided loyalties are common and obvious, for example, between the effect on a career for an unmarried potential donor, or between his or her own family's needs and the needs of the recipient when the potential donor is married. The more cohesive and united the family, the greater the potential for pressures to be brought to bear on individuals. For this reason, we would never contemplate using a donor under the age of legal consent (18 years)—although a few such operations have been done in the USA. We have done few child-to-parent transplants, but even greater pressures—and loyalties—may operate.

Above all, doctors must seek not to add to the already existing pressures on potential donors. In fact, we take a deliberately discouraging stance, and point out to prospective donors all the physical hurdles and tests they must pass before being considered (see below), as well as warning of the possible loss of the graft in honest terms.

Given that someone in the family *does* want to give a kidney, is it reasonable to take that kidney? Putting it bluntly, do the results justify the means, or is a live donor merely a means of getting a guaranteed kidney at a time of choice rather than haphazardly? The operation—which the donor does not need—is not a holiday; it will mean at least a month off work for the donor, two weeks of which will be in hospital, and above all will leave the donor with only one kidney. There is a risk of anaesthetic death of about 1:20 000, and no surgeon is perfect. In a handful of cases, deaths have already occurred in various parts of the world immediately following kidney donation, although I know of none in the UK.

My answer would be that it *is* justified in most cases. The results of live donor grafting remain above those of cadaver grafting over the first 3 years or so, even with the improvement in results which has occurred within the past 5 years. Also, the *really* long-term results—10 years or more—are markedly better. Having an operation of this magnitude carries a negligible risk, and the post-operative discomfort can be relieved. The donor will have the satisfaction, which is not easy to assess, of having helped someone he loves. In addition someone else will be helped: the individual who would now get the cadaver kidney the relative would have needed had they not received a kidney from a relative.

The donor will be acceptable to any insurance company as a normal life with his one kidney, and studies show that within a year or two his remaining kidney will have grown to do the work of two; the risk of injuring it in a motor accident remains, but in statistical terms is trivial. At the moment the very long-term outcome (10 years or more) of losing one kidney is still being studied. It has become clear that some donors do develop high blood pressure and protein in their urine, but the proportion is small; they do not develop failure of their remaining kidney. The donor will be at higher risk of depression in the two years following the graft, and must of course face the possibility that the graft may be one of the few which fail. Every family thinking about a living donor transplant must discuss openly how they might all feel, if the situation arises after two operations, and a sacrifice on the part of the donor, of the kidney having failed and the recipient still being on dialysis.

Blood groups and tissue typing in living donor transplantation   As with cadaver grafts, the blood groups must be compatible before someone can give a kidney, so before anything else the blood group of any potential donor will need to be tested. The different pairs which can be considered are:

Recipient is:	Donor can be:
O	O
A	O, A
B	O, B
AB	O, A, B, AB

From the account of tissue typing given in Box 5, it can be seen that for the HLA A, B, and DR types, fathers and mothers will share half their types with any of their children. Brothers and sisters might be identical (i.e. have inherited the same two sets of types from their parents) (1:4 chance), share half their tissue type (1:2 chance), or be completely different (1:4 chance again). Since matching for even HLA A and B typing seems to make a difference in survival in living donor kidney transplantation, it is worth *selecting* the best donor—if selection is possible—using tissue typing and other tests. Most units are reluctant to do a transplant from a brother or sister who has no tissue types the same as the potential recipient, although we will do this sometimes, for example if there is no alternative, or we know the patient will have to wait a particularly long time for a cadaver kidney.

A possible test here is to do a 'trial transplant' using blood cells from the prospective donor and recipient. The donor's cells are first treated to render them unreactive, then the two are mixed, incubated together and the strength of the recipient's reaction to the prospective donor is measured. This is called a *mixed lymphocyte reaction* (MLR) also called a mixed lymphocyte culture (MLC).

What happens if one is being considered as a kidney donor?   When one plans to go ahead with a willing, ABO blood group, HLA-compatible, MLR-negative donor, there are still many hurdles to be overcome. The first is that when the doctor takes a history and examines you, you must be in first class physical condition, and have a blameless medical history. There is no fixed upper limit of age, but nearly all donors are less than 60–65 years of age. A number of tests will be done to assess the kidneys, as detailed in Chapter 2. He or she must have (of course) two kidneys, which function normally, and clear urine and blood tests. Since a number of kidney diseases are familial, or run in families (see Chapter 3) this may not be a trivial question. We now have a few would-be donors attending our clinic as patients, and at least an occasional would-be donor is known to have ended up later on dialysis themselves! After the orthodox ultrasound, an X-ray of the blood vessels to and from the kidney (a renal arteriogram; see Chapter 2) will be needed to visualize the blood vessels to and from the donor's kidneys, to see that they are normal, and to plan which kidney to take. Variations in the blood vessels to the kidney are quite common, and obviously must be carefully studied. Having passed all these hurdles, one can offer the prospective donor the chance of giving a kidney. On occasion, at this point, he or she will change his or her mind, and it is important that it be seen that this is possible. The actual operation of giving a kidney is described later in this chapter.

Cadaver donor transplantation: where have all the kidneys gone?

First, which unfortunate individuals can be cadaver donors? There are a few exceptions. Patients dying with widespread cancer are not suitable, because the cancer may have invaded the kidney and could be carried over into the recipient with the kidney. Patients who have widespread infection are also unsuitable, for similar reasons: both bacterial and viral infections can be given with the kidney to the recipient. Both these situations are made worse by the immunosuppressive drugs given to the recipient of a kidney graft. Potential donors who have had a very low blood pressure, or severe heart failure are not ideal, but these kidneys will often work very well. However, there is a higher risk of failure, and these are not usually taken. In general, people dying over the age of 65 are not often used, because kidney function declines with age. No one knows, however, whether an 'old' kidney which is transplanted into a young recipient can be 'rejuvenated' to some extent in a young recipient. Sadly, kidneys from children above the age of only about 5 years are excellent, and although small, will rapidly increase in size if transplanted successfully into an adult. However, they are needed especially for small children who require transplants but are too small to take a full-size adult kidney, and these must have preference.

These exclusions still leave us with many suitable kidneys. The 'ideal' donor is the unfortunate young (or middle-aged) person who has had an accident to their brain which has destroyed the possibility of recovery, but who is being maintained on a ventilator to keep him/her breathing. The commonest reason for this tragedy is traffic or other accident; sometimes a bleed from an un-diagnosed blood vessel malformation in the brain may lead to the same state. Many other medical causes of death can lead to this state, but are less common.

The importance of being on a ventilator is that the kidneys are still being perfused with oxygenated blood and functioning well. If the kidneys are taken after the heartbeat and breathing have ceased, they do much less well. If actual death has taken place more than half an hour before the kidneys are taken, and certainly more than one hour, then the kidneys will be damaged beyond repair. The ventilator allows everything to be done without hurry, and give time for relatives to be contacted (see below), and for the possible chances of recovery by the potential donor's brain to be assessed, usually again and again. Nowadays almost all kidneys are taken from individuals who have already died but are being maintained on ventilators, and this is perhaps one of the reasons why results of cadaver kidney transplantation have improved. Fears of patients having their kidneys taken out when they might otherwise have recovered have to be allayed today. It can be said without equivocation that irreversible brain damage *can* be diagnosed with certainty, and that this is *not* a problem.

Every year in the UK, twice as many people die in accidents as die of renal failure, and half of them die on the roads (3800 deaths per year). In the USA in proportion to population more than twice as many die on the roads—more than 50 000 every year. Each person unfortunately dying in this way has *two* kidneys, so that there should be no shortage of donor kidneys. In fact the proportion of donor kidneys that comes from road accidents has declined steadily over the past 20 years as the road death total has fallen. Now, the commonest donor is an unfortunate person who has suffered a major event inside his or her head/usually a bleed or stroke. It is a sad fact that the greater number of people killed on the roads, the greater the number of cadaver transplants done (Figure 25).

The great majority of the public are not opposed to the idea of their organs being used for transplantation, although still in practice about 25-30% of grieving relatives do sometimes exercise their right to refuse. A dozen separate

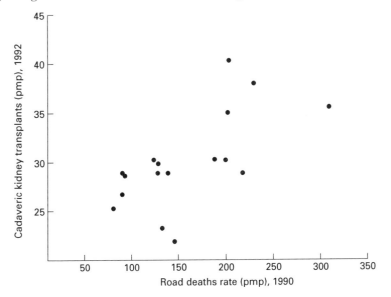

Figure 25   The relationship between the number of cadaver transplants done and the number of road deaths in different countries. (Source: *A question of give and take: improving the supply of donor organs for transplantation.* Edited by Bill New, Michael Solomon, Robert Dingwall, and Jean McHale. King's Fund Institute, London 1994. This small book gives an excellent discussion of the whole problem of increasing organ donor supply.)

surveys in the UK over the past ten years show 75–85 per cent of the public support or are neutral on the idea of organ donation by the recently dead. Even though donor cards are widely available in many countries, including the UK and the USA, still too low a proportion of the population carry them (23%) to have a major impact on the problem. Only 1750 kidney transplants were done in the UK in 1994, but in 1995 more than twice that number (5000) are still waiting for a graft on dialysis—and the total waiting is still on the increase, even though we in Britain still treat only about two-thirds of those that need it by dialysis. The situation is the same in every developed country. In the USA, about 30 000 Americans have functioning grafts, whilst 150 000 are on dialysis. Over 9000 grafts are done each year, but as in the UK, this number needs to double at the least to cope with the need. What is wrong and what can we do about it?

First, how is it that potential donors die in hospital without donation being considered at all? Above all attitudes of individual doctors and nurses are crucial. Unless and until individual doctors at all levels of responsibility see the acquisition of organs for use to help others—and on occasion their own patients—as part of their responsibility we will make little headway. The fault is not with the public, 80 per cent of whom are in favour of donation, and many would argue that no changes in the present laws are needed. However, although the great majority of people say that they support the idea of allowing their relatives to give a kidney, about 30% do not want to give consent when the moment actually comes.

It is easy to see how doctors and nurses who have laboured—or are still labouring—to save a shattered life find it difficult to turn around and treat 'their' patient as a resource. Certainly, patients need have no fears that they will receive less treatment if they are considered to be possible donors; their treatment will be examined and their likely or unlikely prospects of recovery will be examined *even more carefully than usual*. Their task has been made easier by the clear definitions of *brain death*, which have superseded the older obsolete 'cessation of heartbeat and respiration' (both of which can be taken over by machines, if needed). Now the probable prognosis for independent life off a ventilator can be made with accuracy, by testing the functions of the primitive, more automatic part of the brain called the brainstem, by standardized tests. This allows the transplant surgeon to take the kidneys after the diagnosis of brain death has been made but immediately after—or even before—ventilation has been turned off formally, without waiting for all the clinical and electrical activity of the heart to stop.

This raises the questions of the law, and permission to take organs, which naturally varies from country to country. The law governing the taking of tissues in the UK is still the old Human Tissues Act, 1961, which provides a reasonable framework for operation even today, since so much English law is law established by common law practice within a framework of acts of parliament, rather than precisely codified as in Roman law (which, in general, holds in Scotland). In the USA, most states have a uniform donor card backed by legislation. New acts have been suggested, particularly those involving the creation of an 'opting out' system. In this, it would be presumed that any organ could be taken at or after death, unless the individual concerned was carrying some indication to the contrary, or had registered his or her views with a central data bank, to which easy access would be available locally for checking. In fact, such an act has already been introduced in a number of European countries during the 1970s and 1980s, and has been in operation in Scandinavian countries for some time. In France, the impact on numbers of transplants was negligible, whilst in Sweden they remain at a high level. This suggests that factors other than details of legislation determine the rates of transplantation observed in different countries. In fact it is already possible in the UK, under the 1961 Act, to take organs without necessarily seeking permission of the nearest relatives. One practical problem is that it is not clear who the 'nearest relative' may be. By convention, husbands and wives are asked with respect to each other. But what about a widower with several brothers and children?

Even within the present, arguably clumsy framework, the units most active in finding donor kidneys operate at a level which suggests that 2000 or even 3000 kidneys *could* be found nationally in the UK without any change in the present system except better organization. Even 2500 per year would go a long way towards treating the majority of those that need it. Certainly, it would be a useful trigger to the medical and nursing staff if everyone carried a donor card, but the effect will not be great until the majority, rather than a minority as at present, carry such cards. The publicity for donor cards and more recently the donor register also reminds the public—and the medical profession—of the need for organ donation. Transplant Co-ordinators who can devote most of their time to liaison with hospitals in the area of transplant units have been appointed in almost all areas, who in addition can raise the profile of transplantation and have a major educative role. Transferring dying people to intensive care units so that they can be ventilated just for transplant donation was declared contrary to law in 1994 for the UK, in that what is being done is not for the benefit of the patients concerned.

Figure 26 shows transplantation rates in different countries for 1992, and the proportions of those grafts from cadaver and living donors. It can be seen that some countries with the highest rates of transplantation rely much more

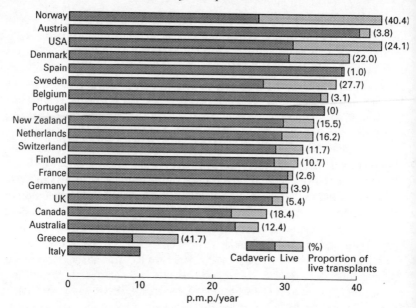

Figure 26 Numbers of transplants done in different developed countries in 1992, and the proportion done from living and cadaver donors. (Source: *A question of give and take*, p. 25.)

heavily on living donors than does the UK: a quarter of all grafts done in the USA are from living donors, and nearly half of those in Norway.

Unrelated living donor kidneys

Today thousands of transplants of this type are being done in the Third World, from donors who are paid, because cadaver donation is not organized (or has hitherto proved very difficult on cultural or religious grounds) and a few individuals have enough money to pay for a kidney. Major ethical problems surround this use of *paid living unrelated donors*. All international nephrological and transplantation societies have condemned the use of such kidneys, and in the UK it is illegal since the passage of an Act of Parliament in 1989, and the European Union has condemned the practice. Others argue, however, that the developed West has no right to dictate ethics to the Third World, but particularly the involvement of Western surgeons or nephrologists in this trade for profit is condemned by almost all observers. India has just outlawed the practice, but in the absence of dialysis for cost reasons the effects of this legislation is unknown.

However, a growing number of *unpaid unrelated live donor* transplants are done today, especially in the USA, from concerned individuals and without payment. The results, initially similar to cadaver donors, now seem to be more like those from related living donors, and the ethical problems this benefit presents are considerable. In this category are husbands and wives, step-parents and long term partners. Few such grafts are being done at the moment, however, outside the USA. For example in Australia in 1992, only 14 such operations were done, 7 wives to husbands, 4 husbands to wives, 2 unrelated but concerned individuals and one adoptive mother. We have used step-parents as donors on two occasions, and have done transplants between spouses.

How long will I have to wait on dialysis for a transplant?

There is really no answer to this question, because it depends on your blood group, whether or not you have antibodies that can interfere with transplantation, and above all whether you have a common or a rare tissue type. Also, it depends on which country you live in. For reasons that are not entirely clear, almost everywhere in the world blood group A patients are quicker to transplant because group A donor kidneys seem to be more frequent than expected; in addition, blood group A patients can have O kidneys as well, whereas group O patients must have O kidneys. The rare AB group is, paradoxically, easier to match, especially since group AB patients can receive kidneys of any blood group, but group B patients may wait a long time in Europe or North America because of the relative rarity of blood group B in the local populations. Finally, if you have antibodies judged to be a problem you may have to wait for a kidney of a specific tissue type, or only a very few types, and this may take years rather than months. This is discussed further in Box 5.

In Britain, during 1984 to 1993, just as the waiting list has increased, so has the average waiting time, from just under a year to a year and three months. Of course the range is enormous—from a few days to ten years or more. However 95 per cent of British recipients on the active waiting list for a transplant can expect to be transplanted within about a year and a half.

Transplants from animals (xenotransplantation)

What about transplants from animals? There has been much written about this in the press recently. In the mid-1960s, several transplants were done from chimpanzees into humans, the longest of which survived a surprising nine months. No further attempts have been made as far as kidney transplants are concerned, although some short-lived, much-discussed liver and heart transplants have been performed, but in the longer term it is probable that xenografts (from the Greek xeno- meaning stranger foreign) will be an important source (see Chapter 11). At the moment there is a great deal of work going on, in the attempt to understand what the barriers are between human recipients and (say) pig donors. Pigs have been particularly favoured as donors, because pig kidneys are very similar to human kidneys in size, shape, and function (see Chapter 11 for more details). At the moment however, non-human kidneys are not a practical option.

What happens if you are to have a transplant?

Probably you will be on some form of dialysis already (see Chapters 6 and 7), although a few patients are transplanted without any prior dialysis, especially if a kidney donor is available within the family. You will already be blood grouped. You will also hear talk about your tissue type which will be determined, as well as any anti-tissue antigen antibodies in your blood which will be studied. Both these topics are dealt with in Box 5 in this chapter.

You will then be put on an active waiting list, until a suitable kidney in terms of blood group and tissue type arises. Different people have to wait very different times to get a suitable transplant (see below), because it is not worth putting kidneys into people which will quickly fail. Not only is this a tragedy for you, but it is also a waste of a kidney which would have done much better in someone else.

During this time of waiting you will be 'on call' 24 hours a day, and may need to inform the hospital of your whereabouts. When a suitable donor is notified, you may have the disappointment of coming to the hospital prepared for the operation, only to find that for some reason the kidneys from the donor were not available or not suitable. This can happen several times to a few unfortunate individuals.

The details of organization vary from unit to unit, but all dialysis patients need a telephone at home so they can be contacted, and it is wise to have an overnight bag packed if you are on call! Also notify any illnesses, such as colds or 'flu, which might interfere with your ability to receive a kidney. After you have been contacted about a possible kidney, it is wise to ask about eating or drinking, since this might delay the anaesthetic.

Will I have to have my 'old' kidneys out?

Not usually, unless they are causing problems, such as infections or pain. If they have to be removed, both kidneys are usually taken out through a cut down the centre of the abdomen, not by one through the side which is used if only one kidney is being removed—for example for a living donor transplant (see below). However in the case of very big and difficult kidneys, as in poly-cystic kidney disease (Chapter 4 and Plate 13), they may be removed one by one. Polycystic kidneys are particularly likely to give rise to trouble, along with kidneys full of stones.

What does the transplant operation involve?

Taking the kidney

The operation of kidney transplantation starts with the removal of the kidney. Clearly this is a different operation if the kidney is being removed from a live donor, or someone who is already dead.

Taking a living donor kidney   What is involved in actually being a donor and giving a kidney? Under a general anaesthetic, the kidney is removed by an operation exactly the same as the one used if the kidney has to be removed because it is diseased in some way, or full of stones. The incision is made in the flank, the kidney is exposed, the blood vessels to and from the kidney are tied and cut, and the ureter tied and cut. The kidney is lifted out of the wound, and flushed with a cold solution (see below), carried into an adjacent operating room in which the recipient is waiting, already anaesthetized and prepared, with the incision made. The kidney is then inserted as described below.

Your side is then sewn up in layers, and you return via the recovery room to the ward. Usually, no drain is needed in or near the wound. The incision can be a painful one afterwards, and injections or infusions of pain-killing drugs will be needed after the operation. Because of the operation and the discomfort, breathing on the side of the operation is shallow and it is difficult to avoid a patch of pneumonia, even if physiotherapy is begun as soon as possible. The donor should be out of bed the next day and home within two weeks. The wound often 'twinges' or gives a 'drawing' sensation for about 3-6 months. Sometimes a small area of numbness is noted on the skin of the abdomen, because small nerves are cut by the incision in your side.

Taking a cadaver kidney   For a *cadaver kidney*, both kidneys are removed, through an incision across the abdomen. They are removed together with their vessels as a single piece, and the two kidneys separated outside the body to ensure good vessels and a good length of ureter. The kidneys are then cooled by flushing them through with a cold sterile solution of salts. The composition of this solution has been worked out by trial and error, but approximates to the composition of the 'soup' within the cells, rather than that which normally bathes them. Each kidney is then placed in a sterile plastic bag of ice.

Kidney preservation and distribution

Prepared like this, the kidney is now safe for up to 24 hours or more. It can be placed within a box and sent by road, rail, or air to wherever a suitable recipient is waiting. The blood group of the donor is needed, and some serum needs to be taken, as well as some cells from the spleen or lymph nodes, to do tissue typing. This can be in progress whilst the kidney rests on ice. Kidney, blood, and nodes will usually be sent or taken all together to the nearest transplant unit, where grouping and tissue-typing (if not already available) is done. The transplant surgeon can then decide whether to use the kidney locally, or send it elsewhere.

There are now a number of national and international organizations for the distribution of kidneys. The United Kingdom Transplant Service is based in Bristol and carries names, addresses, blood groups, and tissue types of the 5000 or so recipients waiting for kidneys all over the country. It also acts as a reference centre for the distribution of reagents for tissue typing, and as a contact with other organizations abroad (Fran Tran-France Transplant; Eurotransplant, based in the Low Countries and Germany; and Scan Tran, in Scandinavia). This 'swapping' of kidneys is particularly important for difficult-to-match patients; that is, those patients with very rare tissue types, and those who have antibodies which render transplantation very hazardous unless a kidney of a particular limited number or type is used, or patients with other special problems.

A considerable amount of work has been done on machines to preserve the kidney for much longer periods than possible with a cold flushing—say up to 72 hours or more. Such machines are now available, but given the rather small distances involved in Britain, and the fact that 24 hours can elapse without problems, even with the simplest preservation, these have not been used much in the UK. However, in other countries, such as Sweden, or in the USA where distances are much greater between centres, the whole transplant programme may be organized around machine kidney preservation. The day when deep-frozen kidneys can be picked out of a deep freeze for use when needed is far off. Kidneys and other organs simply do not recover from this treatment, although the idea is a good one (see Chapter 10).

Putting the kidney in: the operation itself (Figure 27)

You, the recipient of the kidney, will be put in bed and checked over by the doctor; tests will be done to ensure all is well for the operation. The kidney is not placed (as one might expect) in the position of your own kidneys. For this reason, most patients in kidney failure who need transplants do not have their own kidneys removed, although this may be necessary for other reasons. The kidney is put into the pelvis, low down and to one side of the bladder, and the blood vessels of the kidney are joined to the large blood vessels supplying the leg, the end of the artery and vein to and from the kidney being joined to the side of the vessel. The reason for the operation—now almost universal—is the ureter from the kidney to the bladder. It is usually difficult to get a long piece of the ureter, even taking cadaver kidneys, and in live donors it is impossible. Also, one does not want a long piece of ureter, because it then has a precarious

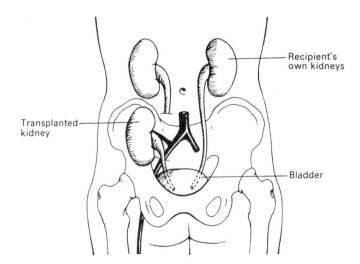

Figure 27 A renal transplant in place. The blood vessels are connected to the major vessels supplying the leg, and the shortened ureter is implanted into the bladder. For simplicity's sake, only the artery is shown, connected to the main (iliac) artery to the leg; and the ureter of the kidney on the side of the transplant has been omitted.

blood supply all the way from the kidney, and may break down from lack of blood supply after the operation. So, given that one uses a short ureter, the reasonable place to put the kidney is in the outer pelvis protected by the hip bone. The kidney lies snugly here away from the intestines and their covering, the peritoneum, and the ureter can be sewn into the bladder.

A minor consequence of this operation is that left kidneys are normally put into the recipient's right side, and vice versa, because of the way the vessels and the ureter lie as they enter and leave the kidney. But this is not essential. The kidney is usually put in the right way up, but occasionally upside down, such as in a few patients who present the problem of having a bladder which has been destroyed or rendered unusable by disease. In this case a new false bladder must be made from a length of small bowel (ileal loop) and the transplanted kidney's ureter put into this.

What happens immediately after the operation?

A kidney transplant is not as major an operation as a heart bypass, or a liver transplant, and you should be out of bed the next day. After only a few days most or all of the various tubes necessary for the operation present in the stomach, into veins, into the bladder—will be removed one by one. Whether the bladder catheter is removed straight away depends upon whether the kidney works immediately (which occurs in almost all live donor transplants, and about two thirds or more of cadaver transplants). If urine is being passed, then the catheter will usually be left in for up to a week. Drains are not usually necessary for the wound, but the intravenous needle may need to be left in for a week or so if you are having infusions of antibodies as part of the medicines to suppress the immune system (see below). Having a transplant is much less painful than giving a kidney, and usually after 24 hours no further pain-killing drugs are needed.

After the operation, a time of stress may be when the graft does not function immediately. This happens in about one third of cadaver kidneys, so is nothing to worry about of itself, and has nothing to do with the final function of the kidney. Some patients will feel that their kidney is 'no good' and this can be a period of great strain on patients and family. This is understandable because of the let-down, after hopes have been raised, and the 'last' dialyses performed. Unfortunately a very few kidneys fail to function altogether, and until urine has been established patient and relatives are under great strain, although the relief of finally getting to the operation may overcome this. The majority of these kidneys pick up in two days to two weeks after the operation, and some of the best kidneys of all in the long term did not work at first. In kidneys which are not working kidney scans (see Chapter 2) will be watched with particular care, and a biopsy (see Chapter 2) of the kidney done to make sure that the kidney looks normal under the microscope.

Most patients also adjust, at least at a superficial level, to the idea of a foreign organ within their body; although most speculate about the nature, and especially the sex of the kidney placed within their body. By and large, it is not the policy of renal units to put recipients and relatives of donors into direct contact, although some on both sides request this. Of course someone who has had a kidney and wishes to say 'thank you' to the donor relatives can write to them, and the unit will pass this letter on through the kidney exchange scheme.

What medicines will I need to take after transplantation?

During the operation and thereafter, all transplant recipients except identical twins will be given drugs to blunt the body's attempt to reject the kidney: prednisolone (Deltacortril, Deltastab, Prednesol), a cortisone-like drug; aza-thioprine (Imuran, Berkaprene), an immunosuppressant drug which interferes with DNA synthesis in rapidly dividing cells, and cyclosporine (Cyclosporin A (Sandimmun, Neoral)). Most commonly all three are given, but any two may be combined successfully and different units use different combinations with about the same results. To begin with, for the first day or two after the trans-plant operation these drugs will be given by intravenous injection, but after 48 hours or so can be taken by mouth. Cyclosporine can be taken dissolved in oil as a liquid, but most people prefer it in the form of large gelatine capsules, though some patients find the capsules difficult to swallow. The longer term problems with these medicines are discussed below.

In addition, many units use infusions of antibody preparations directed against the body's cells which cause and mediate rejection. These preparations of serum or pure antibodies are made in horses, goats, rabbits, and mice (anti-lymphocyte globulin (ALG), anti-thymocyte globulin (ATG), monoclonal antibodies such as OKT3, etc.) and a few individuals react to this foreign protein, particularly if they have had injections from the same animal pre-viously. The infusions are usually given for 7–10 days from the graft, and this means that a neck line (see Chapter 6) or an infusion in the arm must be kept open for this period. If the kidney is already functioning it may delay going home for a day or two.

What is rejection and how is it treated?

The event all transplanted patients fear during the first days or weeks is rejection of the kidney by the immune system of the body. Despite the drugs being given, cells invade the grafted kidney which recognize it as foreign, attack it and are capable of damaging it and if unchecked, destroying it. During the first few months, about two thirds of patients can have rejection episodes, depending upon how well matched the kidney may be, and even those with successful live donor transplants. With the use of cyclosporine, fewer patients now have any rejections, and rejections are fewer in number (usually only one or two at most). The occurrence of rejection episodes is not, of itself, cause for despondency, provided the kidney function returns to previous levels after treatment. Usually, acute rejection episodes become a rare event after only 3 months have gone by. However, this accounts for the very close watch the doctors keep on the kidney—the plasma creatinine and other measures of kidney function (Chapter 2) are done daily or even twice a day to begin with, then after two or three weeks three times a week, and so on, gradually relaxing as the risk of a rejection episode diminishes. The object is to diagnose and treat the episode before it has had a chance to damage the kidney.

Today, most episodes of rejection are treated with three (or more) injections given intravenously of a very high dose of prednisolone (a close relative, methylprednisolone (Solumedrol (R)), is usually given), one on each of three consecutive days. This injection is unpleasant if given too fast, and we usually let the patient control the rate himself after the needle and its plastic tubing have been inserted into the vein by a doctor, or given by pump infusion or a pump syringe. Given too fast, ringing in the ears and flushing may be felt. Alternatively, the daily dose of prednisolone may be increased to a high level temporarily—there does not seem to be any difference in the results, but many doctors feel the methylprednisolone injections have fewer side-effects.

If the rejection episode does not respond to the injections of methylprednisolone, then a second set of three injections may be given. Alternatively, many units will use injections of the same antibody preparations used immediately after the transplant operation in some patients. One preparation is called *ALG (anti-lymphocyte globulin)*, usually made in horses, rabbits, or goats, but use is also made of pure antibodies from mice, directed against not just one cell but against one part of the surface of the cell which is concerned with signalling immune information. One such preparation is called *OKT3*, but many other antibodies of this type are under trial at the moment and will probably play an even bigger role in immunosuppressive treatment in the future.

How will I know if I have rejection?

It can be very easy, but is often difficult! Sometimes you will have a fever, feel
'off colour', and notice that the kidney is tender to pressure. However if you
are taking cyclosporine this is uncommon. The volume of your urine may fall,
and you may gain some weight, and your blood pressure may rise. The concentration of creatinine in the plasma rises (see Chapter 2), and a number of
tests may show changes very early on, which is why so many tests are done
during the first few months, with the aim of catching any rejection episodes
early and nipping them in the bud before any damage can be done to the
kidney.

A transplant biopsy (see Chapter 2), or a fine needle aspiration (FNA), will
often be done at this point. Because the transplanted kidney is at the front it is
biopsied from the front, with the patient lying on his or her back for the test.
A fine needle aspiration is just that—a very thin hair-like needle is pushed into
the graft and some cells from within it sucked out so that they can be examined
under the microscope. Only a very few biopsies can be done, whilst FNAs can
be done daily if needed—but they do not give so much information as a biopsy;
both have a place in helping to diagnose rejection. A principal goal of this
investigation is to decide whether the kidney is suffering from a rejection
episode, or from the toxic effects of too much cyclosporine, or something else—
which is unusual. Sometimes, it is still not clear why a kidney is not doing well,
and arteriograms may be necessary to see if the connection to the artery or vein
is all right (see Chapter 2).

How often will I need to return after I leave hospital?

From one to three weeks on average after the graft, depending on how complicated the course has been, you will leave hospital. By this time you will probably already be feeling the benefit of the operation. Since a lot of the problems
experienced on dialysis relate to anaemia (see Chapters 5 and 6), how much
better you feel will depend upon whether or not you were having EPO whilst
on dialysis. The aches and pains in the joints which some patients on dialysis
experience will usually get better very quickly as part of the side-effects of the
immunosuppressive medicines just discussed, even if the joints are not actually
any better.

Usually you will be seen in the transplant out-patient clinic quite frequently
to begin with—maybe every day, then three times a week, then once a week,

but by the end of the first year or less you will be coming only once a month. The reason for bringing you back is that the risk of graft loss diminishes steadily during the first three months, and then more slowly during the next three months. During this time the dosage of your immunosuppressive drugs wil be 'fine tuned' to give you the maximum benefit with the minimum side-effects. You will need to watch your weight carefully to begin with, just as on dialysis, because to begin with kidney is not too good at regulating this. You may need diuretics, if your ankles swell, or to drink more; some patients find it difficult to drink enough to begin with after long years on dialysis with strict restrictions on intake.

Other medicines you may need include pills to protect the stomach against the effects of the prednisolone, to lower your blood pressure, and to protect you against infections (see below—under complications). Sometimes your phosphate will fall too low—often the sign of a very good kidney—and having spent your time on dialysis trying to get rid of phosphate you now have to eat extra and even take phosphate tablets! Usually the number of different pills you need to take gets smaller with time.

Very soon you will be able to lead a normal life. You will lose any anaemia you may have had on dialysis, and of course will not need EPO because the transplanted kidney will supply a normal amount. Life with a successful transplant is virtually normal except that you need to take medicines and come to the hospital from time to time. Women can think about getting pregnant if they wish, perhaps a year or more after the graft, so long as it is doing well. If you have been transferred from a distant dialysis unit in to the transplant unit, you may well be able to be seen locally in your own unit after 2–3 months, which avoids the long travel which may be necessary for out-patient follow-up.

What complications can I get after transplantation?

Technical complications

Today *technical complications* are rare, but some patients may have problems with leaks of urine from the join between the transplant ureter and the bladder. These usually respond to putting in a catheter for a few weeks, but may need to be operated on. The artery to the kidney may become narrowed at or near the join between the transplant kidney artery and your artery. This is particularly likely to occur when the artery is joined end to end, which is commonly the case in living donor grafts, but it may be seen also is the usual end-to side join normally used for cadaver grafts (Figure 27). Most common, but usually no problem, are collections of lymph fluid around or near the kidney, sometimes discharging to the outside as a clear straw coloured fluid which can look like urine but needs to be distinguished from it. These *lymphocoeles* usually clear up within a few days or weeks, but occasionally have to be drained and closed by a small operation.

Obviously such complications will need investigation by ultrasound, by X-rays of the artery, or cystograms, or by injecting dye into any leak and then taking X-ray pictures. These tests have been described in Chapter 2.

Most of the so-called complications of transplantation, however, in fact relate directly to side-effects of the immunosuppressive medicines you have to take to keep the transplant in place. There is no doubt that these drugs work, but one problem is the side-effects they may produce. Two types of side-effects occur.

Infections

The *first* type is a general consequence of the suppression of immune responses which the drugs produce, and the commonest of these is a predisposition to *infections.* these may occur in any of the common sites—urine, lungs, skin, or (more seriously) in the bloodstream, as deep abscesses, or as infections with unusual germs and other organisms which normally cannot attack a healthy individual. The bigger the doses of drugs used, the greater the likelihood of infections, and now that almost all units use less prednisolone the dangers of infection have receded. However, some infections remain a problem.

One of these infections is the virus called *CMV (cytomegalovirus)*. This is a relation of the chicken pox virus, varicella, which itself can cause problems which I will discuss in a moment. CMV is one of several viruses which can be transmitted in the transplanted kidney, and if you have not had CMV before having the transplant, you are particularly liable to get it from the graft. However it may also recur even if you have had it in the past, since the virus persists in your cells long after the illness has come and gone. Usually CMV infection is rather like a mild influenza, with an intermittent high fever, and feeling off colour. However in some patients it can present as a serious pneumonia. Fortunately we now have drugs which will combat it (gancyclovir (Cymevene), foscarnet (Foscavir)) but understandably CMV is one of several viruses—including hepatitis B and C (see Chapter 5) and the AIDS virus, for which all kidney donors are checked.

Another problem virus is a cousin of CMV, *varicella* the chicken pox virus. This also persists after the attack of chicken pox, usually in childhood, for life in fact. It lives in the nerve roots of the nerves near the spinal cord, and can give rise to the particularly nasty condition of *shingles*, in which the virus travels down the nerve to the skin supplied by the nerve, and causes nasty blisters in a band or stripe. Again we are fortunate in having drugs (aciclovir (Zovirax), famiclovir (Famvir)) which will quickly abort the attack and avoid the often severe pain down the nerve which can persist after shingles.

Yet another virus which once caught, stays with us for life is the *wart virus (papillomavirus)*. The result is attacks of persistent warts following transplantation, on the hands but also on the genitals in some unfortunate subjects. Apart from local treatments such as 'burning' off the wart with very low temperature probes, there is little we can do to help this apart from minimizing the immunosuppressive drugs.

Tumours

Another more worrying side-effect, is a small but definite increase in the tendency to develop malignant growths in the long-term. The reasons for this are not clear: undoubtedly some malignancies (such as *lymphomas*, also called Hodgkin's disease) are caused by viruses which the drugs allow to multiply. In this case the virus is the common glandular fever virus (EB virus). Another virus-related cancer is *carcinoma of the cervix* in women. This is related to a different virus of the same family as the wart virus, (papillomavirus) and it is doubly important for women of all ages who have had a transplant to have at least an annual cervical smear test.

Tumours may be more directly related to the drugs, in that the same mechanisms which reject kidneys 'reject' cancers trying to form, and since the one mechanism is being blunted the other is an inevitable consequence. It must be emphasized that *the risk, although present, is small*. One group of relatively benign growths which are very common after transplantation but which can usually be treated, are *skin growths*. Apart from warts as already mentioned, skin cancers are common, especially in those whose skin is exposed a good deal to the sun, for example in Australia. Thus transplant recipients need to be even more careful than ordinary people not to expose themselves too much to the sun, and to use sunscreens liberally if they do. Also, it follows that most of these skin tumours are in areas normally exposed, such as the face, neck, and hands.

Effects arising from the immunosuppressive medicines

The *second* type of side-effect relates specifically to each drug itself, whether prednisolone, azathioprine, or cyclosporine.

Prednisolone   *Prednisolone* has cortisone-like effects. The most obvious of these, to the patient taking the drug, is the tendency for the cheeks and stomach to increase in size, whilst the arms and legs tend to become thin—an appearance which if extreme has been described as 'a lemon on two matchsticks'. Along with this there is a tendency for weight to increase. How much the face changes is very variable: some patients on bigger doses of prednisolone hardly change at all; others on much smaller doses become very fat in the face. At the same time facial hair increases, and the face becomes flushed. This is sometimes called the 'Cushingoid' face after a Canadian physician who first noted this, in patients producing too much cortisone, from their own adrenal glands.

These changes in appearance can be very distressing, especially to women and above all young girls, given the stress our society places on personal appearance. Fortunately, lowering the dose of prednisolone, which can be achieved if you are taking both other immunosuppressive drugs, results in improvement or disappearance of the problem. Along with the redistribution of fat to the face and abdomen, many patients notice also that they have a voracious appetite, and despite being put on a reducing diet gain large amounts of weight. This may be seen only during the first three months after transplantation, especially if anti-rejection treatment is needed during the early period. For reassurance, it is worth looking at a group of patients who have completed their first year following a graft, or longer. Very few of them have noticeable changes in their faces or bodies.

The other effects are less obvious to you, but may be worrying the doctor more. These include a tendency for the *blood pressure* to rise, a tendency to develop *diabetes* with a high sugar in blood and urine (especially if you have a family history of diabetes), and a risk of developing ulcers in the stomach or duodenum. Your mood and personality may change, not only because of all the tremendous upheaval of renal failure, dialysis, and transplantation, but also as a result of the steroids. This is usually in the direction of a feeling of euphoria and well-being, but very rarely can spill over into mania.

A common problem made worse by prednisolone is thinning of the bones, or *osteoporosis* especially serious in women after the menopause. We do not yet know if hormone replacement therapy with oestrogens (HRT) will prevent or improve this, but studies are underway. Since the loss of bone is very slow, it will take 10-20 years to get the answer. There is no reason why women should not have HRT after the menopause if they wish it, although the dose of cyclosporine may have to be reduced a little. In addition, HRT may be protective against blood vessel disease (see below) and thus would be doubly favourable.

Finally, there is one distressing complication which fortunately is now rare with smaller doses of prednisolone, but very distressing to those who suffer it. This is another bone problem in the joints, especially the hips. This is called *AVN (avascular necrosis)* of the hip, which causes pain on walking. This may be mild but can be intense, persistent, and uncontrolled by analgesics, and the hip may need replacement with a metal one. Fortunately, the results of the operation are excellent, as they are if the condition affects other joints, such as the knee or shoulder.

Azathioprine   The main side-effect of *azathioprine* is depression of the bone marrow, so that the platelet or white cell count of the blood falls; in this case the drug will be stopped for a few days, then restarted at a smaller dose. A few patients have marrow so sensitive they cannot tolerate it at all, and it will have to be stopped. Occasionally, the liver is affected and jaundice appears, and again the drug must be stopped for good.

Cyclosporine   *Cyclosporine* in big doses may give rise to hairiness, trembling of the hands, and an increase in the size of the gums, but all these signs are that the dose is too high and that it must be reduced. The blood concentrations of cyclosporine are watched closely at each out-patient attendance. Its main problem, however, is that it has an *adverse effect on the function of the kidney itself*. This may make the diagnosis of rejection even more difficult in the early days, but is reversible if the dose of cyclosporine is reduced. Doctors have worried about the long-term effects of the drug on the function of the transplant, but current evidence suggests that at the doses used today this risk is absent or negligible.

Blood vessel disease

A final problem which involves a number of factors, some to do with the patient but many to do with the prednisolone and the cyclosporine is an increased incidence of *vascular disease* that is heart attacks (myocardial infarcts), poor blood supply to the legs, and strokes from blood vessel problems within the brain. These are undoubtedly more common in those who have been transplanted than in the general population.

A family history of such problems increases the likelihood of vascular disease, as does having high blood pressure—which many sufferers from kidney failure have had, with or without treatment. Another very strong risk factor is smoking, and to smoke if you have a transplant is playing Russian roulette with plenty of bullets in the gun! There is no reason why transplant patients should not use nicotine chewing gum or nicotine patches. However prednisolone and cyclosporine both affect the final risk factor, which has had a disproportionate amount of publicity: the fats in the blood. Whilst undoubtedly an important factor, the effect of a high blood cholesterol or related fats is much less than that of high blood pressure or smoking. Nevertheless, most transplant units now check the blood cholesterol and fat in their patients with transplants, and if high, start them on a diet which will lower these. If this fails or only partially succeeds, one or another of medicines designed to lower the blood cholesterol and fats will be started. There are a number, and it is not clear yet which is best to use: simvastatin (Zocor), pravastatin (Lipostatin), in the USA, gemfibrozil (Lopid), probucol (Lurselle), Cholestipol, etc.

What can *I* do to avoid the complications of transplantation?

Thus there is a good deal that you can do to avoid the complications of transplantation and its associated medicines. Eat sensibly, taking a diet low in saturated fat and calories; stop or avoid smoking; watch exposure of your skin to the sun; make sure your blood pressure is well controlled by taking your blood pressure tablets regularly; have an annual cervical smear; report any suspicious lumps on your skin early. Above all, don't skip out-patient visits, and take your tablets regularly as prescribed.

Results of transplantation

All this makes transplantation sound pretty dreadful! So it can be, for a patient who loses one or two transplants and suffers many or all of the complications listed into the bargain. However, *for the great majority of patients it offers a virtually normal life*, free of restraints except the need to continue taking pills each day. Let us look at the results of cadaver grafts first, since these are in the majority.

Survival of patients and cadaver grafts

First, the good news is that results of transplantation are improving all the time. Figure 28 shows figures from Britain and Ireland over the past 13 years, and the improvement in graft survival is obvious, although the problem of kidneys being lost after one year still remains about the same.

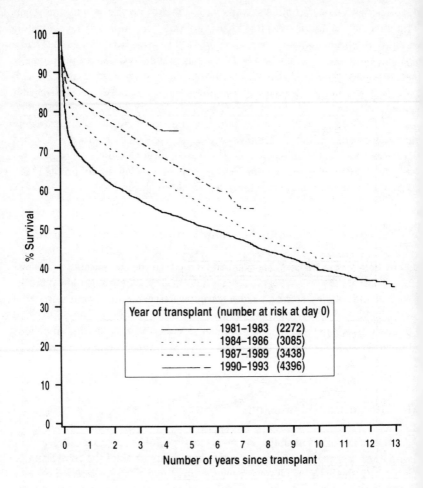

Figure 28 Cadaver graft survival results from the UK and Ireland for 1981 to 1993. The results in the first year have improved steadily over this period, but losses in the second and subsequent years continued at about the same rate. Source: United Kingdom Transplant Support Service Authority: *Renal Transplant Audit*, Bristol, 1995. p. 84.

Next, let us be frank and ask what the risks of your dying during or following a renal transplant may be. More than twenty years ago the results still looked pretty dreadful, and a dialysis patient who accepted the risks of a cadaver transplant was, to some extent, gambling in the hope of a better life. *This is no longer the case.* Better kidneys to transplant, and better use of immunosuppressant medicines, have reduced mortality to very low levels. The risks of dying for a young (under 55 years of age), resilient, well-dialysed patient are thus *very low*—around 0.2–0.3 per cent, that is 2 or 3 chances in a thousand. For patients above the age of 55, and particularly those above 60, the risks *do* rise (Figure 29)—but then they do for dialysis also, and for almost every medical emergency or surgical operation. Therefore older patients need to

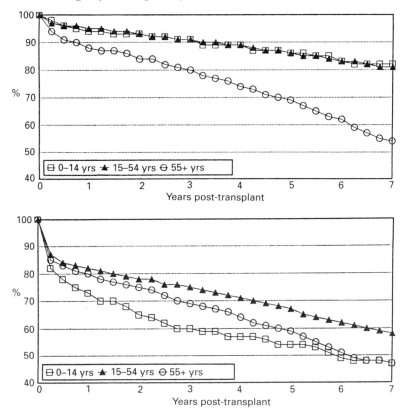

Figure 29 Patient survival (above) and kidney survival (below) following transplantation from the Canadian Organ Replacement Registry, reproduced with permission; data from Europe and the USA are similar. (a) Patients up to the age of 55 years of age have similar survivals, but older patients inevitably survive less well. (b) Graft survival is a little—but only a little—less for older patients than those aged 15–54 years. Of interest is the fact that children aged 1–14 years do not do quite so well over the first five years. This may be because their immune systems are very strong and react more against the kidney. These are average results for graft survival: better tissue type matching makes a difference of about 7% worse (zero match) to 7% better ('full house' 6-antigen match).

consider carefully what the advantages and disadvantages of continuing dialysis may be; for those under 55-60, today there is really no comparison. The results of graft survival will reflect this loss of people with functioning kidneys, and this is shown in data from Canada in Figure 29.

Thus, some transplant surgeons are reluctant to transplant anyone over the age of 55 or 60 years of age. However, now half of the people being treated for kidney failure are over the age of 60. The extra risks of transplantation at this age or greater depends very much on individual circumstances—some patients already have blood vessel disease or even previous infarcts. We do not (as yet) transplant many people over the age of 70, but most have done very well at this age (see Chapter 9). The proportion of the elderly (over 65 years) who receive transplants varies enormously from country to country, from zero in some to 55% in Norway. In the UK the figure is 8% overall, but different units have very different policies on this (see Chapter 9). However the majority of units and countries which offer treatment to this age group, this will usually be some form of dialysis (see Chapter 6 and 7).

Kidney survival: what is the best immunosuppressive regime?

Cyclosporine is undoubtedly successful, but as we have seen above, it is also very difficult to use because of its toxic effects on the kidney—and it is expensive. In our unit, the average cost of cyclosporine alone, after the first few months, was £1400 per year for each patient: that is, its use *doubled* the cost of keeping a transplant patient alive! However, transplantation is still much cheaper in the long run than any form of dialysis, but one of the most expensive ways of treating patients in renal failure is on dialysis after a failed transplant.

It is not clear whether it is better to use cyclosporine alone, or together with a small dose of steroids—or even treatment with *three* drugs in lower dosages: prednisolone, azathioprine, *and* cyclosporine. This in fact is the commonest regime in use today, usually called 'triple therapy'. One would like to get away from prednisolone if possible, because of its many side-effects, but the best results of all seem to be obtainable by some combination of drugs. Also, it may be that the best way to use cyclosporine is only during the first months or year, and then convert to azathioprine. So far, we do not know what the effect of cyclosporine may be beyond 10-15 years.

However, although in cadaver transplantation the *early* results over the first six months or so have improved dramatically with cyclosporine, there is still the same steady loss of kidneys after the first year, as shown in Figures 28 and 29. This is usually the result of what has been called *chronic rejection*, and although it looks very different from acute rejection down the microscope, there is good evidence that it is the result of a slow attack which is based on immune differences, since the loss of kidneys is less when good matching is achieved. It is this effect on long term results which has maintained interest in tissue matching (see Box 5). Also, 'chronic rejection' is commoner in patients who have had several early acute rejection episodes, even when these were successfully treated, than those who never had any rejection episodes.

A number of new anti-rejection medicines are under trial at the moment, and you may be asked to take part in trials of these; they are discussed in Chapter 11.

What causes loss of kidneys?

The great majority of kidneys are lost during the first few months from acute rejection, or after one year from so-called 'chronic rejection' just discussed. A few grafts are lost early because of technical problems, particularly clotting in the artery to the kidney, but this is because of technical problems, particularly clotting in the artery to the kidney, but this is rare. Obviously this is all the more distressing when it happens to a living donor graft. Another rare cause of loss of a transplanted kidney is when the original disease comes back in the graft. This presents obvious problems for the individual affected, but accounts for only about 5% of graft losses in children (see Chapter 9) and only about 1% in adults. In older patients, rejection is less common and less severe, but the number of kidneys lost because the recipient dies incidentally of some other condition becomes greater with increasing age, and more than cancels out this advantage.

Very long-term outlook: late loss of your kidney

However it is a final stress for you if your kidney is found to be slowly failing, when you thought all was going well (see Figure 28). Most patients who have been carefully educated to expect this possibility, and know in detail the odds of success and failure and can cope; but an understandable period of depression and inability to cope with a return to dialysis may follow. By and large, however, it is impressive to see how well most individuals can cope with this major double upheaval in this lives, of hopes raised then dashed.

If a first graft should fail then a second, third, or even a fourth may be put in, with or without an intermediate period back on dialysis, that is the second graft *can* be put in before the first fails (a 'piggyback' graft). Usually the 'old' failed kidney is left in place, unless it gives problems and becomes hot and tender when the immunosuppressive medicines are tapered off. After the second, technical problems may arise because the site which the surgeon would like to use (Figure 27) has already become scarred by the previous kidney. The main problem with second or subsequent grafts however, is sensitization and the appearance of antibodies which render finding a compatible kidney more difficult (see Box 5).

Living donor grafts

For those lucky enough to receive such a kidney from a close relative, the results are very good indeed, with over 90% of people alive and enjoying it 7 years later (Figure 30). How the graft fares depends to some extent upon the exact source of the kidney. A parental kidney, or one with only a half and half (one haplotype) match (see Box 5) do a little worse than those with a full match—which by definition can only be obtained from a brother or sister (see Box 5). Around 80% of these kidneys are still working as long as 15-20 years after (Figure 30). It is unusual to do brother to sister grafts if they do not share *any* tissue antigens (zero haplotype), because the results are no better than with cadaver grafts—but if the situation is desperate, then we would go ahead. Unrelated living kidney grafts do a little better than cadaver grafts, but not so well as a graft from a member of the immediate family.

The position of cyclosporine in *living donor transplantation* is now clear: the 10 year results with cyclosporine are even better than can be achieved with prednisolone or azathioprine, and its use permits the dose of prednisolone to be reduced to negligible levels, or to stop the drug altogether.

Rehabilitation

The *quality of life* with a successful transplant is undoubtedly superior to that on regular dialysis. Most of all, the sense of being tied to the dialysis routine is absent from the transplant life—although it may be replaced with the fear of rejection! Women can and do have children; several have had more than one child, including several in our own unit, and apart from several sets of twins born to transplant recipients, one woman in Glasgow, Scotland had triplets after her transplant! Both men and women can carry on life and jobs relatively uninterrupted. In Europe as a whole 79 per cent of those with functioning living donor transplants were working full-time, and a total of 86 per cent at least part time (Figure 29). Eleven of the remaining 14 per cent were capable of work, but unemployed. Of those with functioning cadaver grafts, 64 per cent were working full time and a total of 76 per cent working at least part time;

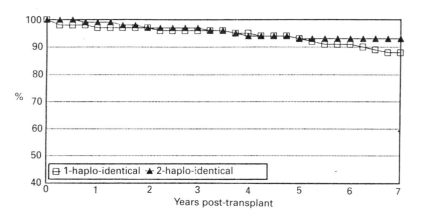

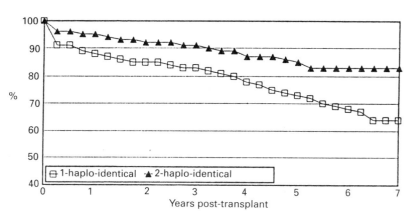

Figure 30   The upper panel gives results from the Canadian Registry, reproduced with permission, for the survival of *related living donor graft recipients* and (below) of the *grafts themselves* (the recipient would normally return to dialysis). Over ninety per cent of those receiving a related living donor graft were alive 7 years later, but in comparing these results with Figure 29 (a) one must remember that the average age of those receiving related living donor grafts was much lower than that for those receiving cadaver grafts. The effect of tissue matching is shown in the lower panel: those who received a brother or sister's kidney with a 'full house' double haplotype (see Box 5) match did better than those receiving a single haplotype match from either a parent, brother, or sister.

19 per cent were capable of work but unemployed; only 5 per cent were incapable of work. In a Europe with 10–15 per cent of the work force out of work, these figures represent excellent rehabilitation.

Conclusions

Transplantation of the kidney has for a long time been an established medical advance rather than an experimental procedure. Looking at the picture overall, for the potentially fatal condition of renal failure, treatment is possible by renal transplantation which results in well over half of all the patients so treated, including those whose grafts may have failed, are not only alive with a successful graft, but' at work or looking after their families full-time. There is little doubt that even these exciting results can be improved (see Chapter 11) and the treatment can, and must, be made available to all who need it. The main problem is to increase the supply of kidneys, both from those who have just died and in the short term from living donors related but perhaps to an increasing extent, unrelated. In cost-effective terms, there can be few (if any) more efficient treatments for a chronic fatal disease.

The UK is doing renal transplants at a rate which compares well with other countries. However, as discussed in Chapter 10, our record of providing dialysis is poor, and we have the greater need to provide more transplantation to compensate for this shortfall. The number of transplants done in the UK each year is no longer rising, and now lies at about 1700–1800 per year. This represents a rate of transplantation of 31 per million population per year (Figure 26), and it is interesting to note that the three comparably sized European countries, France, Italy, and the Federal Republic of Germany achieved 31, only 12, and 34 per million respectively in 1993. In the USA and Australasia, comparable figures are 40 and 27, whilst in Japan as yet little transplantation is done, despite an enormous dialysis programme (see Table 5 for more details).

The reasons for the failure of transplantation to expand to the level needed, perhaps with the exception of the USA and Scandinavian countries (over 35–40 per million per year) varies from country to country. It deserves much more attention, effort, and finance at an international and national level than has been the case previously, if only because transplantation is the most cost-effective way of treating end-stage renal failure.

All these bare statistics conceal, however, the personal stories that make them up. The first child we transplanted more than 28 years ago at the age of 10 lost her father's graft after 5 years, and a subsequent first cadaver graft after 18 years, but had yet another and is now very well and looking after her two growing children. The second ever patient we transplanted still has his kidney 29 years later, helping its owner run a country pub. Living donor grafts are still in place in the USA and France over 30 years later.

9 People with special needs: diabetics, paraplegics, children, and the elderly

The worse the passage, the more we welcome the port

Dr Thomas Fuller: *Gnomologia*, 1732

Facing up to kidney failure is bad enough, but is doubly difficult if, in addition, you have a condition which affects other parts of your body and may have been creating problems for you during many years. In addition, people at the extremes of life—the very young and the very old—have their own special problems.

Diabetes and kidney failure

By far the commonest condition mentioned in Chapters 3 and 4 as causing kidney failure which affects other organs and can cause special problems, is *diaebetes mellitus*. In the USA, 35% of all patients with kidney failure have developed this as a result of diabetes. Both young diabetics who need insulin, and older diabetics who need tablets and diet to help with their diabetes can develop kidney failure.

Exactly why and how this happens is not entirely clear, but the good news already mentioned in Chapter 3 is that certainly in younger diabetics, and probably also in older diabetics, the better the control of the diabetes the less the chance of developing kidney problems. This explains why kidney failure has become less and less common in young diabetics. Fifty years ago, around one half suffered this complication. Now, less than one third do so. Blood sugar monitoring on sticks using a reflectometer at home, as well as divided doses of insulin throughout the day using easier delivery systems such as the insulin pen using pre-loaded cartridges, may have helped—plus of course the efforts of those caring for diabetic patients in better educating diabetics to care for themselves, and of course those with diabetes themselves, have resulted in maintaining better control.

If you are unlucky enough to be one of those diabetics who develops a kidney problem, this usually happens about 15-20 years after you first develop diabetes. If you have already had diabetes for 25 years or more and have not yet had any kidney problems, it is unlikely that you will ever develop them. If you need insulin, it is usually easy to know when your diabetes started. In older diabetics, many people have diabetes for years before it is diagnosed and treated.

The first thing that happens is that *protein (albumin)* becomes detectable in your urine (see Chapter 2). To begin with the amount is very small, too little to detect with the ordinary sticks used to test urine (see Chapter 2), which is called *microalbuminuria*. Later, it slowly increases in amount to become detectable on ordinary stick testing (Plate 2). Eventually it may become great enough to cause the swelling of a nephrotic syndrome (Plate 1), but this is not common.

Your blood pressure tends to rise, and it is *very* important to control this (see Chapter 3). Even so, after 5-10 years at the most, the kidneys slowly fail. Treatment at this point with ACE inhibitors (see Box 1) can slow, and maybe even prevent the deterioration; this is still being studied. Symptoms and signs of kidney failure in diabetics are the same as those in other cases of kidney failure (see Chapter 5).

While kidney failure advances, some diabetics notice that their diabétes surprisingly becomes *easier* to control and they have to back off on their insulin doses. A few people are able to come off insulin altogether! In the meantime, your diabetes and its control will have to be watched with all the usual care. Diet may need to be modified in the direction of a lower protein/phosphate intake (see Chapter 5 for details), and if as often happens high blood pressure is present or appears, salt intake will need to be limited. It can be very complicated having diabetes and kidney failure as well!

Eye problems

In addition diabetics face other complications of their disease. If you have kidney trouble there are between eight and nine chances out of ten that you will have trouble with your eyes (*retinopathy*) or your nerves (*neuropathy*), or sadly, both. The treatment of eye problems in diabetes with kidney failure is the same as for other diabetics. If your eyesight fails because of cataracts in the lens of the eye the lens can be removed and replaced with a plastic one. If the retina at the back of the eye becomes damaged, then laser treatment can help. Treatment of high blood pressure is even more important in limiting damage to the retina. It is a sad fact, however, that despite these treatments your eyesight may fail, and a number of diabetics end up partially sighted or blind; diabetes is the single commonest cause in those registered as blind, both in the

UK and the USA. Obviously you need to have your eyes checked on a regular basis by the ophthalmologist, just as if kidney failure were not present. However, being partially sighted or even completely blind is *not* a reason why you cannot have treatment for kidney failure should you need it.

Neuropathy

Again diabetics with kidney failure often have problems with their nerves as well, and it is not helped by the fact that the nerves are damaged by the uraemia of the kidney failure itself (see Chapter 5). You may not notice the nerve problems at all although the doctor can detect them, but you may have 'burning' feet, hot and cold feelings in the legs, or tingling in the feet. Often all these are worse at night and disturb your sleep. Feet may become numb or feel 'dead'. Occasionally attacks of severe sudden pain occur, but fortunately this is rare. Impotence in men may be a further distressing complaint, as the nerves to the sexual organs are affected. As with the eye and kidney complications, it seems that good control of your diabetes may slow or prevent all these nerve changes, but once they have appeared there is not much that can be done to reverse them, although the symptoms can be relieved in various ways.

Disease of large blood vessels

The problems of the eyes, nerves, and kidneys of people with diabetes are the result of changes in the minute blood vessels within each tissue. However, diabetics are doubly unfortunate in that they may suffer problems in their larger blood vessels much more commonly than the general population. This is particularly so in older diabetics, but may affect diabetics in their thirties and forties. Disease of the large blood vessels to the kidneys themselves may even be a cause of kidney failure in diabetics, as in those without diabetes (see Chapter 3).

How does this come to notice? First, you may get *tightness or pain in your legs on walking*, from narrowing of the main arteries to the legs. The doctor may not be able to feel the pulses in your feet and legs, and an arteriogram (Chapter 2) may be needed to sort out if a block is present, and if so, where it may be. It may be possible to dilate up vessel with a balloon (antioplasty), or use a bypass operation, just as for the artery to the kidneys (see Chapter 3).

The second way blood vessel problems come to light is with *heart troubles*. Specifically, you may notice a tightness or heavy pain in your chest, often down your left or both arms or into your jaw, when you take exercise of any sort. This results from cutting off the blood supply to the heart because of partial blocking of the blood vessels to the heart muscle. Diabetics are much more likely than non-diabetics to suffer this problem, and perhaps to have severe enough narrowing to cause a *myocardial infarct* ('heart attack'). Yet again it may be possible to do a balloon angioplasty or a bypass operation to increase the blood supply to the heart muscle. Some people have quite bad blood supply to their hearts or even a myocardial infarct without recognizing it, and the diagnosis is made by looking at the heart tracing (ECG) or other tests such as heart scans.

Smoking is a major risk factor for large vessel disease in everyone, and above all in diabetics. It is literally suicide to smoke if you are a diabetic with kidney failure.

Problems with feet

These result from a combination of the nerve damage and the blood vessel problems, both large and small. Pain normally protects us from injury, and diabetics with neuropathy lose this protection. Injuries to your feet can go unnoticed, and with the poor blood supply, do not heal. Literally before you know it, an ulcer forms which may be very deep and even involve the bones of the foot.

Thus regular inspection of your feet (see the British Diabetic Association's booklet *Coping with diabetic feet* (Appendix B)), chiropody as needed, and careful selection of shoes are very important. Above all, DON'T cut 'corns' or hard skin off yourself—get a chiropodist to do it for you, especially if your eyesight is poor.

Unfortunately some diabetics have such bad problems with their feet that toes, of even the whole foot, are lost. This emphasizes how important foot care is for people with diabetes.

Can I have dialysis if I have diabetes?

Any form of dialysis can be used where kidney failure is the result of diabetes. In CAPD your insulin dosage and diet may have to be adjusted to cope with the glucose load the bags put into you (see Chapter 7). Usually you will continue to have insulin under the skin, or tablets as before or in modified dose. If your diabetes is 'brittle' and difficult to control diabetes you can inject a much larger dose than usual into the dialysis bag, but this increases the risk of peritonitis and is not used routinely.

One major problem doing CAPD arises if you are partially sighted or blind. Connecting the CAPD bags becomes difficult or impossible by touch alone, and various gadgets such as the UV box are available which help put the tubing together easily and automatically, and you can be taught to use these. In your daily life you are probably managing more complicated things such as cooking, than doing CAPD involves! Totally blind diabetics can do CAPD at home without assistance if they have to and want to.

Haemodialysis presents extra difficulties for diabetics also. Making and maintaining good blood access (a fistula, see Chapter 6) can be more tricky, especially in older diabetics with bad arteries. The surgeon making the fistula has to be very careful in diabetics with poor circulation, to ensure that a cold painful hand does not follow a successful fistula, from blood being diverted up the arm. Blindness does present major difficulties for doing home dialysis yourself, and usually blind diabetics will dialyse in centre, in a satellite unit, or have a partner conduct the dialysis at home.

Can diabetics have kidney transplants?

There are a number of special problems which face diabetics if they are going to have a transplanted kidney. First given the shortage of cadaver kidneys outlined in Chapter 9 many kidney units adopt a policy of not transplanting patients at higher risk. This is in part to protect you, the patient, from the extra risk of problems after the operation, but is directed in part to making the best use of what kidneys are available. Many diabetics unfortunately fall into the 'high risk' category because of heart or blood vessel disease—for example if they have already had a myocardial infarct. Thus, your heart and blood vessels will be examined with especial care and tests done to detect any problems, before a transplant will be considered. The iliac blood vessels to the leg, on to which the transplant is attached (see Chapter 8) may need attention first if they are diseased, or may even prove an impossible barrier to doing a transplant.

In addition diabetics with severe neuropathy may have bladder problems. There is difficulty in emptying the bladder, there is sensation of the bladder being full, and urine left behind acts as a focus for infection. Occasionally it may be necessary for some diabetics to catheterize their bladders regularly to avoid this. Obviously this presents a problem in connecting the new transplanted kidney to the bladder, but you can still have a transplant successfully under these circumstances.

What about a pancreas transplant as well as a kidney?

Double pancreas-kidney transplants are slowly increasing in number, as results improve, but this is still to some extent an experimental treatment. The advantage is of course that you no longer have to take insulin, since the new pancreas takes over. Usually the pancreas is connected to the bladder so that the digestive juices produced by the main part of the gland can pass without harm into the urine, whilst the islets which produce insulin can release this into the blood stream.

Conclusions

Many diabetics in kidney failure have multiple extra problems, besides all the worries of being in kidney failure. On the other hand, people with diabetes hae had to discipline themselves for many years with regard to medicines, diet, and lifestyle, and often are better at coping with the new challenge that kidney failure presents than non-diabetics, as one more difficulty along an arduous road. Choices of treatment may be more limited than for non-diabetics, but many people with diabetes and kidney failure lead full and satisfying lives despite having suffered loss of kidney function.

People with paraplegia

People with paralysis of the legs and lower body (paraplegia) face, of course, many challenges and problems in their lives, related to mobility, continence, and sexual function. In addition however, kidney failure is distressingly common in people with long-term paraplegia, although most escape this complication.

There are two main reasons for paraplegia. The first is that they have been born with *spina bifida (meningomyelocele)* of varying severity. Some have only mild spina bifida, affecting only the very lowest segments of the cord, can walk normally but have some difficulty in passing urine, because the nerves supplying the bladder are not normal. In addition they may have sudden urges to pass urine, which they find difficult or impossible to control ('unstable bladder'). Both can be helped by medicines to control the bladder, but some people in this situation need to do regular catheterization of their bladder to empty it, and can be taught to do this themselves.

More severe spina bifida results in major bladder problems, which along with the useless legs, presents great difficulties. Often the urine will have been diverted by a surgical operation into an artificial bladder created from a loop of small bowel (ileal loop bladder). Today, often a new bladder is fashioned from a piece of large bowel and placed where the normal bladder would be (caeco-cystoplasty), which drains out through the urethra rather than an artificial opening in the side which drains into a bag, which has to be worn permanently;

clearly a better solution, although a larger operation is needed. Sometimes the urethra also may need to be operated on (urethroplasty) with or without a mechanical device to allow continence and control of urine.

The second group of patients with paraplegia are those who develop it as a result of trauma, accidents to the spinal cord (*spinal cord injury*). Occasionally, infections, tumours, or other diseases of the cord produce the same result—a bladder without its normal nerve supply which empties without control, and poorly, often at high pressure. The level of the injury to the spinal cord varies from high in the chest to lower down the back. Treatment is the same as for patients with spina bifida: catheterization, diversion, or caecocystoplasty.

Why do people with spina bifida or paraplegia develop kidney failure?

The treatment outlined above should help to prevent spina bifida patients going into kidney failure, but unhappily there are still people with spina bifida or traumatic paraplegia who have or develop renal failure. This results mainly from *infection* and *obstruction* (see Chapter 3) both of which are treatable and avoidable in theory, but this is not always achieved. Even ileal loop bladders can be infected, develop stones, become obstructed, and the kidneys may be damaged. Usually the kidney failure, if it comes, develops very slowly.

The second problem that paraplegics and people with spina bifida face is *pressure sores*. Because the bottom is numb, as are the legs, injuries are not noticed, nor is the discomfort of sitting too long in one position which presses the blood out of the skin and tissues bearing the weight of the upper body. The skin reddens, swells, and breaks down. At this stage the process can be reversed easily, but if the skin breaks altogether, a large ulcer can form very quickly, which may heal but will need to be exposed without any weight on it, or even plastic surgery.

Chronically infected sores, together with infected urinary tracts, can lead to *amyloidosis* (see Chapter 4). This is regrettably common in paraplegics, and can cause kidney failure.

Can I be treated for kidney failure if I have paraplegia?

The answer is of course yes, but special problems arise. For example, CAPD (Chapter 7) is rarely possible because often the abdomen has been operated on to produce an ileal loop or caecoplasty. If this is not the case, then CAPD can be considered as usual—for example if the ureters drain directly to the skin outside the peritoneum into a bag. However for the majority of paraplegics haemodialysis is the best form of dialysis. Some paraplegics or spina bifida patients dialyse themselves at home, if they have enough support.

Transplantation obviously carries extra complications also, which will vary from person to person according to the exact status of your urinary tract, bladder, or drainage system. First, it may be necessary to take out your old kidneys if they are badly infected, perhaps leaving an ileal loop bladder in place if there is one present. Often the transplant will be attached to this, having positioned the kidney carefully to achieve this. Often the kidney is put in higher up than usual, and sometimes it has to be put in upside down to make a good fit with the ureter! In this position, kidney biopsy (see Chapters 2 and 8) may be difficult or impossible, should one be needed after the transplantation.

Obviously the extra burden of kidney failure as well as all the problems of having paraplegia is difficult to cope with, and you will need all the support you can get from family, friends, and the kidney unit staff, especially the social worker. On the other hand, by the time you do come to kidney failure, you will have proved already, to others and yourself, that you can face adversity with success.

Children

Obviously, children face extra problems if they should be unlucky enough to develop kidney failure. Childhood is a time of growth and development, not only physical but also in terms of personality, emotional make-up, and relating to other people. All of these may be interrupted, slowed, or diverted by kidney failure and also by its treatments, however successful.

What causes kidney failure in children?

The principal causes of kidney failure are a little different from those in adults. The predominant group of children with kidney failure are born with kidney problems, or develop them early in life. The commonest cause is *reflux* of urine into the kidneys, and if this happens before the child is born, the kidneys may not develop properly (*dysplasia*). Reflux is especially damaging if in addition there is obstruction to urine outflow and a high pressure within the urinary tract (see Chapter 3 for discussion).

The next main group is *inherited disorders* such as *Alport's syndrome*, *cystic kidneys*, *oxalosis*, and *cystinosis*. All of these are discussed in Chapter 4, except cystinosis which is discussed in Chapter 3. Finally, a minority of children with a *haemolytic-uraemic syndrome (HUS)* do not recover kidney function. This again is discussed in Chapter 4.

Forms of *glomerulonephritis* are the next most common cause. The child may be find until 5–15 years of age, when one form or another of the *nephrotic syndrome* (see Chapters 3 and 4), or of acute nephritis appears. As mentioned in Chapter 3, many children get over either of these problems on their own, or can be treated, but a minority have ongoing diseases in which kidney failure develops. Principal types are *FGS (focal glomerulosclerosis)* and *MCGN* (see Chapters 3 and 4).

Does kidney failure have special effects in children?

As mentioned above, the principal extra effects are on your child's physical and emotional growth. Children in kidney failure may grow poorly, and rapidly fall behind their classmates. They may be deeply disturbed by hospital attendance and treatments. Bone problems are more common in children than in adults with kidney failure.

Can anything be done about all this?

The principal route of help is through good nutrition, and control of blood phosphate levels (see Chapters 2 and 5). Kidney failure diminishes appetite, and left to themselves many uraemic children become very 'picky' and simply do not eat enough for growth. The dietician can help to increase and balance your child's intake of food, and help to make meals more palatable in the face of diminishing appetite. To control the blood phosphate, phosphate binders will be needed (see Chapter 5), and children often need treatment with vitamin D (see Chapter 5).

Also, recombinant (genetically engineered) growth hormone is safe and very effective in promoting growth in height in children with kidney failure. The main problem is its high cost—about £20 000 ($30 000) each year for each child at the moment in the UK.

What happens when end-stage kidney failure is reached?

A plan must be made for each child in the short and the long term. In the short term, dialysis is usually necessary, although if a kidney is available from a parent (see below) then transplantation can sometimes be done without any dialysis being necessary.

Both haemodialysis (Chapter 6) and CAPD (Chapter 7) can be done in children as young as 1 year, or even in newborns, although CAPD in the form of APD, or overnight PD, is much easier in tiny infants. If haemodialysis is to be temporary, for only a few months, then a subclavian line (see Chapter 6) or a haemocath external line may be implanted for access. This can be opened to connect to the dialyser. Special small dialysers (artificial kidneys) and low volume tubing is used in small children. Haemodialysis is rarely done at home in children, because although feasible the disruption of the home and disturbance to other children in the family renders it traumatic for all.

For CAPD small size CAPD catheters are available, and the exchange volumes are of course smaller also. Otherwise CAPD in children is just the same as in adults; older children can do their own exchanges which allows them the freedom to attend school and be at home, which is a big advantage. Obviously, smaller children must be helped by a parent, visiting nurse, or unit staff whilst in hospital.

Whilst your child is maintained by dialysis of either type, nutrition will be of great importance in keeping bones healthy and promoting growth. If all else fails, again growth hormone can be effective.

What about transplantation? Can any child be transplanted?

General aspects of transplantation are discussed in detail in Chapter 8. There are no absolute reasons why any child in kidney failure cannot be transplanted. In practice however, it is very difficult and has a very high complication rate under about 10 kg (20 lb) in weight—size is more important than age, since many infants in kidney failure are smaller than they should be at their age. Thus dialysis may be done until the infant is big enough to have a kidney transplant successfully. Most paediatricians see transplantation as the major goal in treating end-stage kidney failure in children and adolescents, even though dialysis can if needed maintain reasonable health throughout childhood. Bladder problems increase the difficulty of transplantation, but hardly ever make it impossible.

Where do kidneys for children come from?

Like adults, children can receive *cadaver* kidneys (Chapter 8). Surprisingly small children of 10–20 kg (20–40 pounds) can be transplanted using adult kidneys, but the majority of children receive a kidney from a donor aged less than 16 years. Especially in small children and infants, these kidneys are, sadly, ideal for children on dialysis, and are used when available. Children are put on the waiting list for a transplant kidney alongside the adults, but get 'first refusal' on kidneys from donors aged less than 16 years.

However, most parents will want to consider whether or not to give a kidney to their child. The whole question of living donor transplantation is discussed in Chapter 8. A parent who wishes to give a kidney must be an appropriate blood group for their child (see Chapter 8), must be perfectly fit with two normal kidneys. The main question however is how parents feel this sacrifice will impact on their own relationships both with their partner and with other children in the family, or future children. Pregnancy is of course possible with only one kidney. In some families however, for example if the child is a rare blood group in the West such as blood group B, or has major problems with antibodies (see Box 5) then a parental kidney may offer the only way out. Paediatric kidney units differ very much on their attitude to parents giving kidneys, and this will need to be discussed with the unit staff. Occasionally older brothers or sisters are suitable, but in the UK must be over 18 years of age to be able to donate.

Is the operation any different from that in adults?

In general no, but in very small children it may be necessary to connect the blood vessels of the kidney to the main blood vessels, the aorta (the main artery), and the vena cava (the principal vein), rather than to the somewhat smaller vessels running down to the leg (see Figure 27). The ureter of the kidney is placed as usual into the bladder. The management, complications, and medicines used are essentially the same as in adults, and are outlined in Chapter 8. The drug cyclosporine may make your child hairier than before, and a few children develop coarser features on this drug. If this happens then alternatives may be sought or the dose reduced.

What about growth after transplantation?

Usually this is better than in kidney failure or on dialysis, but depends critically on the amount of prednisolone given, since this retards growth. The doctors will attempt to use as little as possible, and it will often be given every alternate day rather than daily, because this seems to help growth.

Will my child's activities be restricted after transplantation?

Apart from sensible precautions because of vulnerability to infections, especially in the early days after the graft, the answer is that there are almost no restrictions. Contact and other sports in which the kidney might be damaged by a blow are best avoided, such as rugby, karate, or trampolining. Otherwise the whole aim of transplantation is to return your child to a normal life.

Immunizations are probably less effective than in normal children, because of the immunosuppressive medicines (see Chapter 8), but should still be given. However, a vaccination with a *living* virus or germ must be avoided: these include oral polio vaccine (the injection form is safe), measles, BCG, and (if you are going abroad to an affected area) yellow fever. Exposure to chicken pox can be a problem, because it can spread alarmingly, and your child may need an injection of globulin (antibodies) for protection, and you should let the unit know if exposure has occurred.

The elderly

Elderly patients have many extra challenges should they enter kidney failure. In addition, they form the largest group of patients requiring treatment for end-stage kidney failure.

How common is kidney failure in the elderly?

End-stage kidney disease is a disease principally affecting the elderly, as we saw in Chapter 3. Table 2 illustrates this fact, from figures on how many people at different ages in the population have end-stage kidney failure in the UK, and Figure 31 shows the same for those actually under treatment for kidney failure in the USA; there is almost twice as much kidney failure in the USA as in England. To begin with only younger patients were accepted for treatment, but now that in almost all developed countries all patients are considered for

Table 2 New patients each year of end-stage kidney failure in the United Kingdom by age

Age (years)	New patients/million people/year
0–19	6
10–49	58
50–59	160
60–69	282
70–79	503
80–	588

Study of Feest and colleagues in Manchester and Devon. *British Medical Journal* (1990). **301**, 987–90.

treatment if they have end-stage kidney failure, the dominance of the elderly is clear.

The average of those under treatment is now above 60 years in both Europe and America, which of course means that *half those needing treatment for kidney failure are aged more than 60*; in some countries such as Sweden, the average is already over 65 years, and the commonest single group in the USA is 65–70. In some other patients such as Afro-Americans and Afro-Caribbeans, the incidence is even higher amongst the elderly, mainly related to the frequency of non-insulin requiring diabetes in these groups.

Why is kidney failure so common in the elderly?

The principal causes of kidney failure in the elderly are diabetes, disease of the blood vessels to the kidney (see Chapter 4), some glomerulonephritis, polycystic kidneys, but in many old who develop end-stage kidney disease we

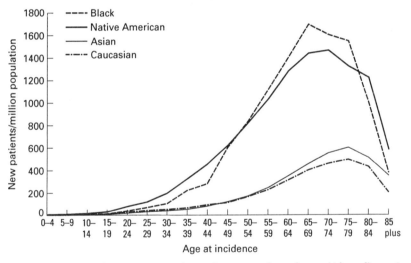

Figure 31 Ages of patients on any form of treatment for end-stage kidney disease in the USA in 1991 (Source: US Renal Data System). The numbers rise steadily from childhood to about 65–75 years of age, and then fall sharply. This fall represents the small number of very elderly people (over 80–90) but also the fact that, at that age, a smaller proportion of people actually get treatment should they develop kidney failure. Note also that the numbers of people requiring treatment are much greater (2.5:1) in the Afro-American and Native American groups than in Asian or Caucasian (white) population. This accounts for the greater numbers of people requiring treatment for kidney failure in the USA than in Europe; the same is seen in Afro-Caribbeans living in Britain.

simply do not know why they go into kidney failure. Kidney function falls steadily from the age of 25 years or so, and by the age of 130—if we lived that long—almost everyone would be in kidney failure! It may be that a proportion of those elderly with kidney failure represent simply a rate of decline in kidney function which is faster than that of other organs.

Moreover, the number of elderly people in Western populations has increased enormously, and is still increasing, which multiplies further the numbers of elderly in renal failure. Although many more people survive today to an advanced age, the absolute limits for age have probably not changed: the number of centenarians in the UK has gone up tenfold from 200 to 2000, but the oldest Briton ever remains at 115 years, and only 1 in 100 million lives to be 110 years. Nowadays, the 60s are regarded as middle age, and 'elderly' refers to those over 70 or 75 years of age.

Centenarians themselves have varied opinions as to why they have been spared for so long: Fanny Thomas aged 113, said 'eat apple sauce three times a day and never marry'; Mrs Divi Bastoulemos of Barbados, aged 112, recommended 'plenty of sex, plenty of sun, plenty to drink, no work and no children'. In contrast, in Scotland Mary Neilson, 106, reported that 'I dinna smoke, I dinna drink and I dinna go wi' men'. On the subject of diet, American junk dealer Richard Lewis who died aged 105 smoked ten cigars a day and is alleged to have drunk one or two bottles of Thunderbird every day. Every week he consumed about 2 kg (4 lbs) of sugar in his drinks, a dozen eggs, pounds of streaky bacon, and a family sized tub of fried chicken! However, the most important single factor is genetic: the long lived have long lived children. The best recipe for a long life is to pick your ancestors carefully!

People in general, including those looking after patients in kidney failure, are often ignorant of just how much longer an elderly individual may be expected to live. Table 3 shows figures from the USA, but the UK figures are similar. Note that someone aged as much as 75 years could ordinarily expect to live until the age of 85 or 86: we must not use conservative treatment as a cheap way of neglecting to treat our elderly patients.

Special problems in older patients

If you are old you have a number of physical, psychological, and social problems to overcome. In the *physical* field, eyesight may fade, coordination be poor, mobility difficult, hands arthritic, memory erratic for recent events, and dexterity reduced. Malnutrition of various types is frequent even in the non-dialysed elderly, for a variety of reasons varying from attitude and choice, through immobility to frank poverty. Other organs besides the kidney deterior-

Table 3   Estimated survival at different ages of the USA population in 1986

| At age (years) | White men | | White women | |
	Life expectancy	Expected age at death	Life expectancy	Expected age at death
60–	18.2	78.2	22.6	82.6
65–	14.8	79.8	18.7	78.7
70–	11.7	81.7	15.1	85.1
75–	9.1	84.7	11.8	86.8
80–	6.9	86.9	8.8	88.8
85–	5.1	90.1	6.4	91.4

Data for non-white US citizens are slightly inferior from 60–70 years, and slightly superior thereafter.

ate with age, and poor and variable output from the heart and rigid blood vessels present major problems.

In the *psychological* field, many elderly people lack goals in their lives, suffer intermittent depression, and find it difficult to face up to the major challenge of survival in kidney failure, especially in achieving self-care using some form of dialysis at home.

Socially many old people are often separated from their families who have grown up and left, suffer from isolation, and lack support if things go wrong. However in some elderly people treatment for chronic kidney failure actually provides them with a clear goal in life, and a 'club' to which they belong in the dialysis unit and which provides them with the contacts they lack in ordinary life. Many elderly people are amongst the poor, relative to the standard of living in their countries; in many European countries the prolonged recession and the high cost of social services has resulted in deliberate or concealed cuts in finance supporting the elderly. Fewer and fewer younger individuals in work support a growing army of the old.

Should every older patient in end-stage kidney failure be treated?

One major, very important difference between the young and the elderly is the fact that whilst young populations are relatively homogenous in their (usually good) health, the normal elderly vary widely, from robust good health on the one hand to complete mental and physical decrepitude on the other; their 'biological' age may be much greater or much less than the number of years they have lived. Thus a strong argument can be put for the view that no patient should ever be excluded from treatment on the grounds of chronological age alone.

In every country a number of elderly patients in end-stage kidney failure still do not receive any treatment—even in countries with supposedly comprehensive services for kidney failure. The majority of these patients today are 75 or 80 years of age and above. The complex reasons for non-treatment, appropriate or not appropriate according to opinion, have been much debated, and we will say a little more about selection of people for treatment later.

Are there *any* absolute features which would always make one turn down a particular elderly patient in kidney failure for treatment? Here we raise some very controversial issues. Whilst one can take the attitude that every individual in renal failure should be given a chance, and treatment withdrawn if life becomes impossible, in the real world budgets simply do not permit this attitude in many countries. In addition, a slow 'death by treatment' may be terrible cruelty. Most doctors pay more attention to mental and physical state than actual age, and would not take on patients even in the early stages of dementia, or with major mental illness. In general, patients with advanced cancers would not be treated, but many patients with early or treated malignant disease are taken on. Otherwise almost no physical factors render dialysis impossible. The real question is whether the person will benefit enough for a long enough time to justify treatment.

What treatments are best for elderly patients?

As in the treatment of ESRD as a whole, there is no one 'best buy' (see Chapter 10); the object is to try and identify, for each individual patient, what is the best mode of treatment for you, given your unique circumstnaces. How older patients are treated in different countries varies a great deal (Figure 32).

Centre haemodialysis has been—and remains—overwhelmingly the predominant mode of treatment for elderly patients in end-stage kidney failure in Europe and the USA. Is this justified? One big advantage is that you can *receive* dialysis in this setting, rather than having to attempt self care, which for many older folk is no longer possible. This loss of independence is compensated for by the security centre dialysis gives, and the feeling of a 'club', mentioned above, is particularly strong. One problem is lack of mobility complicated by poverty, and transport to and from the unit is often necessary.

Haemodialysis presents many problems for older people, however. An unstable circulation from myocardial disease and decreased flexibility of the circulation may lead to difficulties in fluid removal during dialysis, without distressing sharp drops in blood pressure, and in the opposite direction minor degrees of fluid overload lead to severe congestion in the lungs. Irregular heartbeats may be a problem also. All these can be minimized by using dialysis with bicarbonate and careful profiling of fluid removal, or using longer slow dialysis. However these problems may prove insuperable, and make haemodialysis impossible for you. Ultra-short dialysis regimes are bad for older patients, and American data have shown us recently that there is not only an increase in problems, but an actual increase in the death rate when these techniques are pushed to the limit in elderly patients.

CAPD has great advantages for the elderly, and this treatment is common in countries such as Britain and Canada, where it forms the major form of treatment used in elderly patients. The treatment is kind to the cardiovascular system, although patients with poor heart function may have to maintain their weight very strictly within narrow limits (often called 'windows') of 1 kg (2 lbs) or even less. To do CAPD however, you need reasonable eyesight and reasonable dexterity with your hands: if you have a tremor of arthritis, CAPD may be impossible. Yet again, nutrition is vital, and some elderly patients on CAPD may have poorer nutritional state than younger patients, despite the extra energy provided by the glucose in the dialysate. The glucose load may bring out a tendency to diabetes common in older people.

You and your doctors can choose between the two forms of dialysis on an individual basis: survival figures and time spent in hospital in elderly patients in general do not differ much between CAPD and haemodialysis.

Is dialysis in very old patients worthwhile? What is the *quality* of this extended life? Some studies from the UK have shown *better* life satisfaction in patients over 60 on dialysis than younger patients, whilst some American studies have painted a gloomier picture: 40% of dialysed patients over 60 spent all day in a bed or chair at home, and almost half reported some symptoms of depression. However, life was viewed as 'very satisfying' or 'satisfying' by 55% of the respondents even in these studies.

What about *transplantation*? In many countries the elderly are *never* considered as transplant recipients; in some countries few patients over 60 or even 55 years are considered. Figures from the USA showed that in 1988 the proportion of patients with transplanted kidneys falls steadily with age (Table 4).

By contrast in some other countries, such as Norway (Figure 32) the elderly are regarded in the same way as younger potential recipients: who is right? In general, in almost all countries younger patients are given preference. This probably arises from a feeling that older patients are not strong enough to withstand transplantation, that they will suffer more frequent complications,

Table 4 Patients under treatment for end-stage kidney failure in the USA December 31 1988 and 1985 (Figures for Europe are similar)

Age (years)	On dialysis	With transplant	Total	% with transplant	
				1988	(1985)
0–19	1 863	2 328	4 191	55.6	(46.8*)
20–44	29 194	23 020	52 221	44.1	(35.7*)
45–64	46 668	14 198	60 867	23.3	(12.3)
65–74	29 360	1 216	30 568	4.0	(1.5)
75–	15 172	50	15 222	0.3	(0.1)

* In the 1985 data the age groups are 0–14 and 15–45 years.

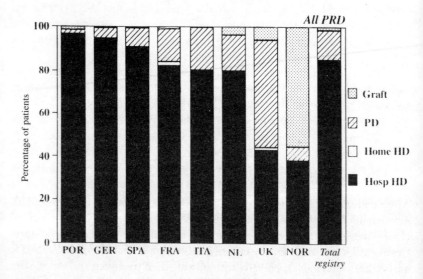

Figure 32 Treatment received by people aged more than 65 years of age when they develop end-stage kidney failure in different European countries. In some, such as Germany and Portugal, almost all patients are offered haemodialysis (HD), almost always in a dialysis or satellite centre Hosp. In contrast, in Britain much greater use is made of peritoneal dialysis (PD) at home, and uniquely in Norway older patients are transplanted just as frequently as younger ones. Data of the European Renal Association.

but above all that they will not survive long enough to 'justify' the use of precious donor kidneys, which are in short supply all over the world, and likely to remain so until xenotransplantation becomes a clinical possibility (see Chapters 8 and 11). However, the figures for expected survival of elderly people (Table 3) do not provide justification of *themselves* for exclusion of older people from receiving a renal transplant, until they have reached an age of at least 70 years. Obviously, patient survival—and hence graft survival—becomes worse with age. This is mainly the result of blood vessel problems, whilst surprisingly cancers play little part. The continued shortage of cadaver organs has led to examination of the use of older *living* donors for older recipients. This approach has received little attention outside Norway, where surprisingly good results have been obtained, and this practice is likely to expand. In fact the results in the elderly are only a little worse than in younger patients, because although in the elderly kidneys are lost whilst still working because their recipient dies, older people reject kidneys less frequently because their immune system is more feeble than in the young.

Do older transplant recipients have the same medicines as younger ones?

Rather gentle immunosuppression must be used for elderly recipients, because the immune system in the elderly is less efficient than in younger recipients, and rejection episodes are less frequent the older the recipient.

When is it justified to stop dialysis?

More and more frequently as we attempt dialysis in progressively more frail elderly patients, or adopt a 'trial of dialysis' to avoid the ethical problems of choice, we simply transfer the problems down the line. Every person who starts treatment for end-stage kidney failure needs to know that the option exists, if life becomes intolerable, of quietly withdrawing from treatment and waiting the inevitable consequences. Much more difficult is when the patient themselves becomes incapable of deciding, because of dementia. Then the burden of deciding what to do falls on their family and the renal unit team; this is never an easy thing to do, or to manage with dignity. Neither inappropriate law nor litigation should interfere with an already difficult situation, but both problems can arise.

Conclusions

It would be sad to end this section on such a gloomy note, because the majority of elderly patients enjoy the chance to extend their lives and watch their grandchildren and children grow, and participate in activities of their choice. Nevertheless, we can never forget the many practical and ethical problems that treating very elderly people with life supporting treatment brings up.

10 An overview of treatments for kidney failure

There were, at the end of 1992, just under 600 000 people being maintained by some form of dialysis, and about 200 000 people with functioning transplanted kidneys. Thus in the next year or two the number of people alive who would otherwise have died will exceed one million. Which form of treatment is best? Of course there is no answer to this question, because it depends entirely upon what individual people want, and what may be best for them medically.

Who should receive which treatment?

One problem faced by most patients with kidney failure is: which treatment should I have, at least to begin with? Of course for some people choice is limited or non-existent, for example previous operations may make CAPD impossible (see Chapter 7) or strong antibodies make transplantation very difficult (see Chapter 8). However most people have some room for decision on this.

Thus we can now choose between home haemodialysis, satellite unit haemodialysis, in-centre haemodialysis, CAPD, APD at home or in hospital, haemofiltration, and transplantation. It is pleasant to have so many choices for a condition which was not so long ago universally fatal in a few days or weeks. The choice will be determined by several factors:

(1) your preference, and that of your family;

(2) the availability of services locally;

(3) the renal staff's reading of the situation;

(4) the availability of a suitable kidney for transplantation.

It may be that after thinking about one form of treatment as first choice everyone will change their mind—for example, after circumstances change, or if a live donor of a kidney becomes available in the family, or if you cannot manage the training for home dialysis or CAPD. The important fact is that *the different treatments should be seen as complementary to each other*, and not as antagonistic; and that the choice of first treatment is just that, with no implication that this will be the *only* way you will be managed for ever.

In fact most patients pass through several forms of treatment, depending on circumstances and success achieved.

How can I choose?

Together with discussions with the renal unit staff, meeting patients who have already been through the whole business, and having an actual look at the hardware you can build up an idea of how you feel about the various treatments.

In practice, a kidney transplant straight off before your kidneys finally fail—perhaps the best solution—is only possible if a donor is available within your family. Thus most people will have to make a choice between one form of dialysis and another to begin with.

Many factors will go towards determining how you feel about different forms of dialysis. Some people find the idea of a rubber tube in their abdomen disgusting and repellant, others make nothing of it. Some hate the idea and the fact of having needles stuck in their arm, others push them in themselves without trouble. Some people want to look after themselves at home, whilst others feel the need for the security of being looked after in the unit. Some prefer haemodialysis because it gives at least some days when you can forget about the whole business, whilst others like the better mobility CAPD can give. If you are at work or looking after a family, this may have a major impact on your choice. The survival of people with either form of dialysis is the same (Figure 33) but *technical problems* are much commoner with CAPD, which means that a number of people on this form of treatment have to change to haemodialysis, and only between a third and one half are still using it after 5 years (Figure 33).

Will I get a free choice?

In many countries, including the UK, financial and even political factors regretably may influence which treatment can be recommended for a particular patient. For example, in the UK at the moment there is a shortage of places for in-centre dialysis, whilst self-dialysis at home is well developed. The number and distribution of satellite or local centres also remains grossly deficient, although this deficiency is being tackled actively as I write. Thus some people

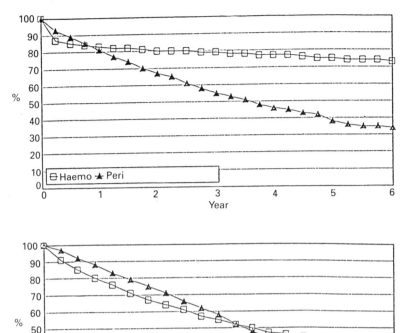

Figure 33 Data from Canada comparing survival of people having haemodialysis or peritoneal dialysis. The top panel shows that the technique of haemodialysis is much more robust, that is you can continue doing it successfully more often than for CAPD, in which only 60% of people who start off doing this are still doing it at the end of 6 years. However in terms of how well you will do, as shown in the lower panel there is nothing to choose between the two. Data courtesy of the Canadian Organ Replacement Registry for 1992.

who would rather be having in-centre dialysis may be pressured to have CAPD or home haemodialysis. Automated machine PD (APD) at night is not available as it should be either, principally because it is a very costly form of treatment. (Finances and costs are discussed later in this chapter.) The solutions to these problems are financial, political, and organizational, not medical.

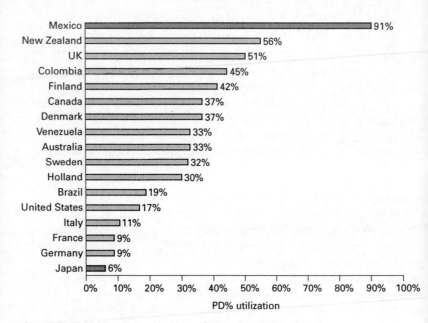

Source: Renal Division, Baxter Healthcare Corporation, 1993 (estimate).

Figure 34 The different proportion of people doing haemodialysis and CAPD in different countries. Despite—or perhaps because of—the fact that there is little to choose in terms of outcome between the two techniques, different countries choose very different patterns of treatment for people in end-stage kidney failure.

In some countries such as Mexico, more than 90% of dialysis patients have this in the form of CAPD (Figure 34), whilst at the other extreme some countries such as Japan have less than 10% on this treatment, almost all being on in-centre haemodialysis. In Portugal (not shown in the figure) only 3% of patients on dialysis receive it in the form of CAPD! As Chapter 8 indicates, transplant rates vary enormously not only between countries (see also Table 5 below) but within different regions of the UK. Figure 35 shows the differences between countries in which treatment patients with kidney failure are having—independently from differences in absolute numbers of people receiving treatment. Unfortunately, it must be said that in some countries, doctors' incomes

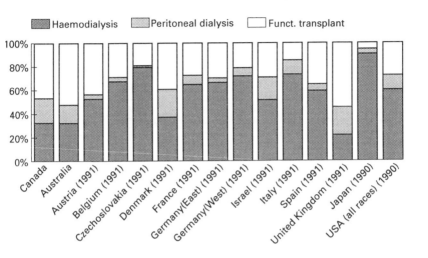

Figure 35 The different proportions of people in renal failure receiving various treatments in different countries in 1992. Courtesy of the Canadian Organ Replacement Register.

depend upon a large number of patients on haemodialysis, and as a result few patients are offered the possibility of CAPD or of transplantation as they should. Obviously, this practice must be condemned.

People with some diseases present special problems, for example diabetics (see Chapter 9). Treating the kidney failure does not help the diabetes itself, and may even make it worse. Also, the other complications of diabetes are in general not affected by successful treatment of kidney failure. Thus a diabetic may face the problem of losing his or her sight after having had dialysis, or a successful kidney transplant, or have severe problems with circulation to the feet, or suffer a heart attack. The outcome for the kidney in transplantation in diabetic patients are nearly as good as those in non-diabetics.

Can I have a transplant?

Many doctors feel that the risks of transplantation, which rise with age, are too great to permit regular transplantation in patients over the age of 60 or 65 years (see Chapters 8 and 9 for more discussion). This mirrors reactions to taking patients in the early days of dialysis, and probably cannot be defended very far. In fact, successful transplants can be performed with a reasonably low risk in patients up to 75 years of age, or even more. However, most doctors working in nephrology feel that older patients are in general better candidates particularly for CAPD, or home, limited-care, or centre haemodialysis. The real problem is the lack of cadaver donor kidneys—we simply do not have enough kidneys to give to everyone quickly. This is discussed more in the next section.

At the other end of life, detailed studies have shown that whilst home dialysis is feasible in children under the age of 15, the strain on the families (and on the other children in particular) is great. Also, growth is poor on dialysis, poorer than in children after successful transplantation. Most pediatricians, therefore, regard transplantation as the best treatment for children, and reserve long-term dialysis in children and adolescents for those who, for immunological reasons, have rejected one or more grafted kidneys.

Thus the choice of treatment for kidney failure is not a simple matter. Many factors, medical and social, will have to be taken into account.

Allocation of kidneys

The whole question of how kidneys for transplantation, which remain in short supply, are or should be allocated remains a subject for heated debate. A mixture of social pressures, medical factors such as age or blood vessel disease, and how many kidneys may be available all play a part. How much attention should one pay to tissue matching, which undoubtedly improves results, and how much to how long the patients have waited for a kidney? Is it better to have a kidney which will last 20 years after waiting 5 years, or one which will last 10 years, after waiting only two years? There are no easy answers to these questions.

Most units put some, but not all, of their patients on call for transplant. Those excluded are particularly elderly and frail patients, or those with complicated diseases. Persistent infection may not allow the use of the immunosuppressive drugs needed for the transplant (see Chapter 8). A particular problem is people—often adolescents or young people—who find it difficult or impossible to stick to the discipline of the treatments involved. Many doctors feel that a kidney is so valuable that they cannot afford to risk losing the kidney because the recipient does not take their immunosuppressive tablets.

Those who are on the transplant list will have all their medical, psychological, and social factors considered when a possible kidney comes up which matches them and several others. Who to give a kidney to is always a difficult decision for the renal unit staff, and understandably many people feel they are being discriminated against, when in fact it may simply be that no suitable kidney has come up (see Chapter 8 for details). In some units, the data are fed into a computer and a program decides who should have the kidney. One advantage is that the computer, although necessarily limited by the data programmed into it, is unbiased at the point of decision!

What are the overall results of treatment for kidney failure?
(Figure 36)

We have discussed in previous chapters the outcomes following different *treatments*; what matters in real life, of course, is what happens to *you as an individual*, whatever treatment you may have after starting treatment; many people will go through two, three, or four different modes of treatment, perhaps ending up back on some form of dialysis. Everyone entering on some new venture wants to know what their chances of success may be. This is obviously true of someone taking the fairly dramatic step of beginning treatment for end-stage kidney failure. However a precise answer for each individual is not so easy to give.

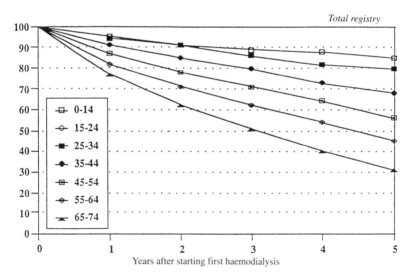

Figure 36 Survival of all patients known to the European registry from 1986 to 1991 over the next five years (any or all forms of treatment). A marked effect of age at the beginning of treatment is seen, with older patients surviving relatively less.

Also, the results of any treatment can be looked at in two ways: first of all, *how many* patients who would otherwise have died survive with treatment? In the case of end-stage kidney failure without treatment *all* would rapidly die, so any success is a significant gain. The second aspect of outcome, much more difficult to measure, is the *quality* of the life achieved.

Figure 35 gives the overall survival of all patients—more than 150 000—in Europe who started any treatment for end-stage kidney disease over a five year period from 1986 to 1991. Clearly, one problem is that obviously everyone does not have the same chances when they start on a treatment programme for end-stage kidney disease. Some are young, and some are old: no-one expects the survival of a 60- or 70-year old to be the same as a 20-year old. The figure shows the effect of age. Some have just got kidney problems, others diseases affecting many other parts of the body (see Chapters 3 and 9).

Also, when comparing results of different treatments, allowances must be made for the different mix of patients who receive that particular treatment. For example, patients who receive kidney transplants tend to be younger and fitter than those who remain on dialysis. Many older patients who have poor heart function, or diabetics, may be directed towards CAPD as their favoured treatment because it is relatively kind to the heart compared with haemodialysis, and the risks of a kidney transplant may be too great. Thus to compare results for transplantation with CAPD directly would be nonsense.

With all forms of treatment the young do better than the old, although the very young (under 5 years of age) do worse as well. Even allowing for age however, no group of patients do as well as their contemporaries without kidney failure, especially in the USA and above all in elderly patients and this is something doctors are still struggling to eliminate. Diabetic patients and those with blood vessel disease as a cause of their kidney failure do less well than those with other forms of kidney failure.

Thus, survival using regular dialysis averages 70 per cent at 5 years after starting treatment for patients on home dialysis, and about 10 per cent less for hospital dialysis. The better survival of patients on home haemodialysis is partly the result of selecting the most robust and competent patients for this form of treatment. Survival in the young is better than in the old, as might be expected. Survival at 5 years of patients on home dialysis throughout Europe varied from 81 per cent for those aged between 15 and 34 years at the time treatment started, to 73, 62, and 58 per cent for those aged 35–44, 45–54, and 55–64 years respectively.

Patients using CAPD have a very similar outlook and thus there is little to choose between these two forms of treatment in terms of success, as already mentioned (Figure 33). Although patients who are transplanted survive better than patients on any form of dialysis, much of this difference is the result of selection of fitter patients for this form of treatment, but some is the result of it being intrinsically a better form of treatment.

Quality of life

Survival is not, of course, the only criterion of success in the evaluation of any treatment. The *quality* of your life is equally important, and in economic terms, your ability to return to productive work, study, or look after others such as your family, or to enjoy an active retirement. Here again, detailed study of these points has been made for people treated by both dialysis or transplantation.

It is much more difficult to measure how good the quality of someone's life may be, although standard questionnaires have been developed to try and do this. It is much easier to assess the work status of people under treatment, if they are over 20 and less than 60–65 years of age (Figure 37). On this

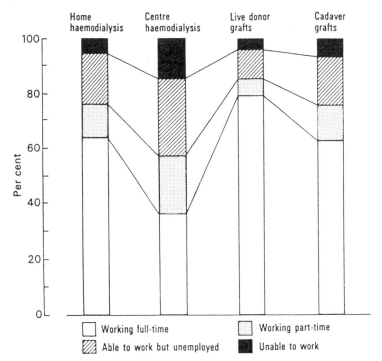

Figure 37   Rehabilitation of patients in Europe receiving different forms of treatment for end-stage kidney failure (see text).

criterion, of the dialysis techniques, home haemodialysis scores better than in-centre haemodialysis, because the dialysis schedule can be modified to suit work, caring for a family, or school. Some patients dialyse in the evenings and on Saturdays; others three times a week overnight. Of home dialysis patients in Europe, 64 per cent are in full-time work and 76 per cent in some work. Another 18 per cent could work, but are unemployed or better off on Social Security. Given present rates of unemployment in Europe, this is a very good performance. Hospital dialysis patients fare worse, partly because many have to dialyse in hospital during the day; in this group, 37 per cent are in full-time work and 57 per cent in some work. Twenty nine per cent could work, but are unemployed. Thus, only 5 per cent of home dialysis and 15 per cent of hospital dialysis patients are unable to work at all. Figures for patients having CAPD are about the same as for home haemodialysis.

The need and the provision (Table 5)

The UK   In developed Western countries many estimates of the number of patients needing treatment for end-stage kidney failure have appeared. Some countries appear to have more kidney failure than others, such as the USA (see below). In Britain, of the 7000 going into end-stage kidney disease each year (134/million total population/year), about 5000 are aged less than 80, and 1800 less than 45 at their deaths. In 1992, 3731 new patients were treated for end-stage renal failure in the whole UK (Table 5). Probably, nearer 5000 (80/million/year) should be treated if the need is to be met for all those under 80 years of age without other serious disabilities and a likely good quality of life, and the British government accepted in 1993 that the National Health Service should struggle to achieve this goal as soon as possible. Take-on rates in Wales already exceed 100/million/year for a predominantly Caucasian population.

If patients up to the age of about 60 are considered, the performance of British renal failure units matches those of the rest of Europe and North America and exceeds the performance of many European countries for transplantation see Chapter 8). It is for those *over the age of 65*, and for *older diabetics* that the British services fail to cope. The inevitably poorer results in terms of survival in these older patients, with or without diabetes—although still better than the treatment of many diseases whose costs are never questioned—plus the feeling that the loss of a 60- or 65-year old represents a lesser depletion of society than a 35-year old, presumably led to the acceptance of this relative neglect by the British medical profession and public alike. The ethics of

Table 5 Rates of take-on for treatment of end-stage kidney failure in the developed world[a]

	Population (millions)	New patients taken on for treatment of end-stage disease (per million people/year)	Total number of patients having treatment for end-stage kidney disease (per million)	Number of kidney transplants done each year (per million)	Number of people with kidney transplants (per million)
Large countries (population more than 50 million)					
Japan	123.6	157	810	6	41
USA	249.4	132	758	40	271
UK	57.4	62	388	30.5	209
Germany	78.0[b]	70 (94)	356 (439)	22 (31)	89 (95)
Italy	57.6	59	503	10	116
France	56.4	64	505	31	204
Medium sized countries (11–50 million)					
Canada	27.4	98	519	27.5	243
Australia	17.5	61	403	27	211
Spain	39.4	60	569	38	210
Benlux[c]	26.0	68	572	34	219
Nordic[d]	23.9	69	285	36.5	293
Small countries (population 10 million or less)					
New Zealand	3.4	69	388	34	
Israel	4.6	106	545	25	156
Austria	7.7	105	460	41	201
Portugal	10.3	86	365	35	117

[a] Sources: national registries and EDTA-ERA; data are almost all for 1992, with some data from 1991 and updated in a few instances to 1993.
[b] Former West Germany had much higher rates (in brackets), and former East Germany much lower rates, than these figures for the new united Germany.
[c] The Netherlands, Luxembourg, and Belgium.
[d] Norway, Sweden, Denmark, and Finland.

allowing someone to die of a treatable condition, who has contributed throughout his working life to a scheme designed to protect, because he or she is now retired and contributes nothing in financial terms, does not bear examination. Although the British government has stated that no-one should be denied any treatment on grounds of age alone, in fact many factors operate to ensure that the elderly, and especially the very elderly, do not receive comparable treatment to those younger than themselves. Several instances have received publicity recently, and the public has justifiably been outraged.

Britain still spends a lower proportion of its national income (gross national product or GNP per person) on health care compared with other Western nations: around 6 per cent in 1991 (Figure 38). In comparison, most other Western countries such as France, Germany, Sweden, etc. spend a larger proportion of their higher income on health, from 7% up to 10%. Although the new structures of the Health Service brought in since 1990 have greatly increased administration costs (from 6% to about 11% of the total spent) the money spent upon the British National Health Service is still spent more

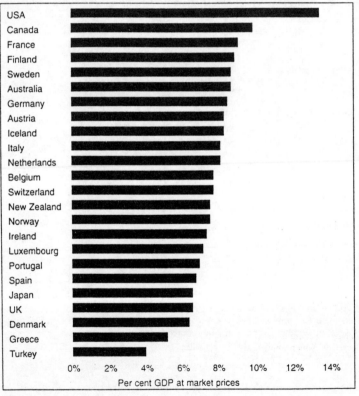

Note: *Figures include public and private expenditure.
Source: OECD.

Figure 38 The proportion of national income (Gross National Product, GNP) spent on health care in various developed countries.

efficiently than in most other health care systems in Europe or in the USA, where the overheads reach around 25%. However, all purchasers of Health Care (District Health Authorities and Consortia in England) have an enormous number of demands on their money, of which kidney failure is only one example; on average only about 1.4 per cent of their overall budget is spent on kidney failure. However, dialysis and transplantation are life-saving treatments, and again the government has agreed that it should be available to all who can benefit from it. The problem is in assessing who might be better off not receiving it, with the inevitable consequences (see Chapter 9); most of the patients will be over 75–80 years of age.

We must also examine whether treating patients in end-stage renal failure is really so expensive, and what it costs to let them die—a question far less frequently asked. It is difficult to cost any aspect of health care with certainty. Both dialysis and transplantation have been analysed more carefully than many other areas of medical practice, on an international basis. Inflation and different costs of living in different countries make absolute figures rapidly obsolete, but the best estimates of the total annual cost (i.e. materials, staffing, supporting services, and depreciation on buildings) for a patient in the UK at 1993 prices are shown in Table 6.

Table 6 Basic costs of various forms of treatment for end-stage renal disease in the UK

Treatment	First year (£ per year)	Subsequent years (£ per year)
Home haemodialysis	31 000*	23 600
Centre haemodialysis	29 140	29 140
CAPD	17 520	17 520
Transplantation without CyA	12 500	3 570
Transplantation with CyA	21 000	4 000

* Includes costs of approximately £8000 for capital equipment (dialyser, etc.). CyA, use of cyclosporine, which improves results (see Chapter 8).

To some extent these detailed financial comparisons are spurious, and depend very much on how patient costs are assessed and allocated; they are to give a general idea only. These costs include hospital admissions, which are very variable with age, underlying disease, other complicating conditions, etc. and so cannot easily be averaged. Comparative costs also vary with the renal unit policy on when a patient with CAPD peritonitis should be admitted to hospital. To begin with, most units admitted most people with peritonitis; now few admit any but the very ill, as confidence in dealing with this complication has increased. Finally, these figures are basic costs and do not include disconnect CAPD systems, or the use of EPO.

In addition, there are a number of so-called 'quality issues' which do not improve survival, but have a major impact on the quality of life. Erythropoietin (EPO) (see Chapters 5 to 7) is an example. It can transform how a patient on dialysis feels and performs, but does not affect survival as far as we can see. However it will add £3000–£5000 each year to the cost of dialysis. Machine APD may suit particular patients much better than CAPD, but costs about £8000 per year more than standard CAPD. Even within CAPD, the disconnect systems which allow you to take the bag off and not carry it around cost about £3000 a year more than the standard bag which stays connected.

It is obvious that successful transplantation offers the cheapest treatment over a period of several years, and that of the several modes of dialysis, in-centre dialysis is the most expensive, and home haemodialysis or CAPD the cheaper alternatives.

At the moment (1996) services for renal failure in the UK probably cost about £300 million per annum—about the same as four medium-sized airliners, or a couple of frigates for the Navy. At the beginning of 1993, this £300 million paid for treatment of a total of 22 300 patients on treatment in the UK, 10 300 on dialysis and 12 000 with successful kidney transplants. In 1992, just under 4000 new patients were taken on for treatment (65/million total population), and 1750 kidney transplants were performed.

It is important when thinking about the costs of a kidney failure programme to realize that *it costs more and more money each year simply to continue taking on new patients at the same rate*—until the rate of exit by death equals the intake. With the population such as is taken on to treatment in the United Kingdom, this will take well into the twenty-first century! If the intake rate is to *increase*—which everyone, including successive governments has agreed it should—then this will require *more* funds—probably about £400–£500 million per year at 1993 prices. At equilibrium, we can estimate that some 45–50 000 people will be receiving treatment for end-stage kidney failure in the UK, with almost 6000 new patients being taken on each year.

All these figures assume that the best survival at present attained is achieved; it is a melancholy fact that the cheapest patient is a dead one—provided only he or she does not consume too many resources in dying. This single fact immediately pin-points the impossibility of adequately reconciling cost-effectiveness with total care; any solution is bound to be a compromise, and the argument is what level of service is acceptable: ethically, practically, and politically.

The USA   In the USA, it has become apparent that kidney failure is commoner than in Europe. Estimates suggest a figure of about 60 000 Americans die of renal failure each year (240 per million total population). Why this high rate? Many factors are probably involved, but two which are now recognized are: first, a higher incidence of diabetes and of renal failure from diabetic kidney disease in the USA, and second, a very high incidence of kidney failure in Americans of predominantly African origin, mainly the result of severe high blood pressure and diabetes, and not from nephritis or other primary kidney disease (see Chapter 5 and Figure 31). Figure 31 shows just how much higher the rate of kidney failure is in black Americans, as well as in native Americans and those of mixed Hispanic/native American blood. Recently, the federal government has launched a $52 million initiative to investigate the management of high blood pressure in Afro-Americans.

As well as providing the most comprehensive dialysis facilities in the world, except perhaps for Japan, the USA makes good use of transplantation (Table 7), with a greater number of living donors than most countries (see Chapter 8). Nevertheless, as everywhere in the world the number of transplants has ceased to rise at an annual rate of just under 10 000–40 per million population per year, 24% of which are from living donors, and the waiting list for grafts is rising steadily, reaching 26 000 in 1993.

As to provision of health care and treatment for kidney failure, a contrasting economic problem has presented itself, compared with Britain. Health costs in the USA have run virtually out of control, with overheads over 25% of the 13% or more of the GNP spent on health, whilst nearly 40 million poorer Americans have no health cover at all. In recent years, the US Government led by President Clinton attempted to introduce new structures for health care provision, but this failed. Nevertheless, *some* action to contain health costs and make delivery of health care more efficient has become essential.

In 1972, after only a brief debate and without detailed forward costings, the Senate passed into law a proposition (public law 92-03) permitting funding of treatment for end-stage kidney failure for all those who might need it. Funding of renal failure treatment in the USA is on a national basis, depending upon the number of patients treated or dialyses performed, although the number of dollars paid to the unit for each dialysis has been reduced steadily over many years.

Costs of treating kidney failure in the USA are higher than those in the UK—an average of $47 000 per year, taking all patients and all patient costs together, irrespective of treatment. At 1993 prices, the basic cost of in-centre dialysis was about $55 000 per year. The American end-stage renal disease programme cost only $242 million in 1977, but rose to $851 million in 1979, $1.4 billion in 1981 and during the 1980s and early 1990 soared to over $5 billion per year. It has now reached $8.6 billion at 1994 prices—about two and a half times bigger than the British figure at equilibrium (£500 million or $750 million), allowing for the difference in populations of the two countries—the United States has over four times the population of the UK. By the end of 1995, over 200 000 Americans were receiving treatment for end-stage kidney failure, and approaching 30 000 new patients started treatment each year. Probably at equilibrium more than a quarter of a million Americans will be receiving treatment!

These figures have led to much debate in the USA as to how costs can be limited without denying treatment. Similar projections to those already given for the United Kingdom suggest that the USA is approaching equilibrium for treatment of patients up to 75 years of age, and that numbers of patients under treatment will depend upon the proportion of those in the ninth and tenth decades of life who receive treatment. Clearly, these people will inevitably be frail, have many other coincident medical problems, and equally will inevitably have a rapid turnover, and will affect the total numbers in the 'pool' requiring treatment at any one time to a much smaller extent than younger patients.

Canada Canada has a well developed health care system which many feel is an ideal compromise between total state provision and personal insurance. In 1992, 14 211 Canadians were under treatment, 6664 with a functioning transplant and 7547 on dialysis. Of these, 37% were using CAPD, perhaps because many of the currently used techniques for CAPD were first used in Canada. In 1992, 755 transplants were done, and (as in most western countries) this number is no longer increasing, and the waiting list for a graft had reached 1823 by the end of 1992.

The financial dilemma

It is clear that neither locally-determined 'rationing' of treatment as in the UK, or the completely open door, as practised in the USA, offers the ideal alternative. In particular, the quality of life and degree of rehabilitation of some very aged demented or severely damaged patients on centre haemodialysis leaves much to be desired; but experience has shown that outcome in individual elderly patients is almost impossible to predict. Treatment of some 'difficult' groups (such as older diabetics) is still far too low in the UK.

In the UK 'rationing' of treatment in older patients still operates mainly at the level of low expectations on the part of patients and their families, together with failure of family practitioners and general physicians to refer older patients or those with other problems to already overloaded units. Thus the actual

Table 7

	£
Long-stay hospital/nursing home care:	
Geriatric	23 500 per year
Mental handicap	18 000 per year
Prison	
Average	22 000 per year
High-security	ca 40 800 per year

(1993 prices. *Sources*: DoH; HM Government)

providers of treatment in the Renal Units have to make 'life or death' decisions much less frequently than is supposed.

The costs of treatment for end-stage kidney disease discussed above sound alarming, but must be looked at in the context of other expenditures which are rarely, if ever, questioned. Let us examine the costs, in the UK, of some other chronic forms of care (Table 7). It becomes difficult to question money spent on maintaining the life of an otherwise fit, sane, law-abiding, productive individual, in the light of these figures. Further we need to consider the costs, in financial terms at least, of allowing patients with terminal renal failure to die. This is obviously more difficult to estimate, and will vary greatly. For example, allowing a retired person of 66 to die will cost little; a young adult with a family will cost a great deal more, whilst losing a child is apparently cheap, but loses the valuable asset of a future wage-earner and potential skilled person. One careful estimate of the cost to the state of losing a 25-year-old man with a wife and two children, produced during the 1980 discussion of heart transplants by the London *Sunday Times*, put the loss to the state at £30 000 (£120 000 at 1993 prices) over the first four years alone. A figure of some £50 000 (£200 000 at 1993 prices) as the total cost of losing a 50-year-old man was also suggested.

In completing this analysis we must also ask just how much other surgical and medical procedures cost per patient, and whether the investment in these is justified in terms of results. A comparison of *survival figures* for some common diseases is revealing, but fewer good estimates of the cost of treating them are available (Figure 39). Attempts have been made to compare the *costs* of both quantity and quality of life, and one such attempt is the 'QUALY', or quality-adjusted extra year of survival. There are many potential and actual

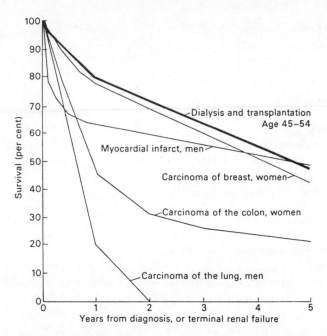

Figure 39 Survival of middle-aged patients on dialysis and transplantation compared with survival from other common medical conditions. (The survival data for the renal patients are for the whole of Europe, for the other conditions from the UK.) (Sources: Registrar General's reports, EDTA-European Renal Association.)

flaws in the calculation of such figures, but for interest Table 8 compares the cost of a single 'QUALY' using different treatments for different conditions. As expected, transplantation again shows up much better in this analysis than dialysis, emphasizing the crucial need to expand this form of treatment through a better supply of kidneys, from whatever source.

Conclusions

Despite the relatively poor quality of life, the time spent on the procedures, and the failure to reverse many of the complications of uraemia, regular haemodialysis and peritoneal dialysis provide an extraordinarily successful palliation for end-stage kidney failure. It is true that they to some extent merely prolong the problem, but useful survival can be attained by most patients in both

Table 8 Cost of a 'QUALY' at 1990-1 prices in the UK

Intervention	£
Cholesterol testing and diet treatment (age 40-59)	220
Neurosurgery for head injury	240
Putting in a heart pacemaker	1100
Hip replacement	1180
Heart bypass operation, severe angina, left main	2090
Kidney transplant	**4710**
Breast cancer screening	5780
Heart transplant	7840
Cholesterol testing/diet treatment (age 25-39)	14 150
Haemodialysis at home	**17 260**
Heart bypass operation, mild angina, one vessel	18 830
CAPD	**19 870**
In-centre hospital haemodialysis	**21 970**
EPO treatment (say 10% reduction in mortality)	**54 380**
Neurosurgery for malignant brain tumours	107 780

(Source: Mason, J. *et al.* (1993) *BMJ*, **306**, 570-2.)

human and economic terms. For some, it is the preferable treatment. The alternative treatment, transplantation, is undoubtedly more successful in terms of rehabilitation, as well as being the cheapest option.

11 *The future*

The only way to predict the future is to have power to shape the future

Eric Hoffer: *The passionate state of mind*, p. 78, 1956, Secker and Warburg.

Attempting to predict the future is always a faulty exercise, since the greatest changes are wrought by events, ideas, and especially techniques which are unforeseen, and often unforeseeable. Progress in medicine, which is an art based upon science, always arises from a combination of ideas and techniques. Both transplantation and dialysis are examples of ideas which were present long before the techniques to make them practicable became available (see Boxes 3 and 4 in Chapters 6 and 8). Finally, even when both ideas and technique are present, practical, financial, or political difficulties may stand in the way of application. However, the greatest barrier to progress is often that health professionals are unable to unwilling to see things in a new light, or to behave in a new way. Thus progress may sometimes have to await a change in generations.

I will only consider here, therefore, the near or immediate future and deal with those ideas and techniques which are already current in thinking or in the laboratory and likely to be applied in the clinic within the next 10 years.

Prevention of kidney failure

It is safe to predict that our capacity to avoid kidney failure will increase in the next ten years. First, we are beginning to understand more about the genesis of *high blood pressure* and especially the genetic factors which lead to its appearance. Very soon it should be possible to screen individuals or the population to identify those at especial risk for high blood pressure and its consequences, especially kidney damage, by examining their DNA for particular forms or mutations of genes coding for renin and other substances concerned with the appearance of high blood pressure. New families of medicines to lower the blood pressure are in the pipeline, as well as newer versions of some old friends which are equally or more effective but have fewer or no side-effects. For example, medicines which block the binding of angiotensin to its receptor are already available such as losartan (Lozaar), and may be in wide use in the near future.

However, it must be realized that the main defect in preventing kidney failure arising from high blood pressure is that treatments already available do not benefit those who need it, because of side-effects or insufficient education of the patient. Without creating a nation obsessed with its blood pressure, screening is now widespread and has already led to early treatment in many who a few years ago would not have been detected, before damage could occur. The salt in the diet of the population as a whole has gone down in most developed countries, and this too should help.

Obviously also the 'new genetics' based on DNA technology must help us in dealing with inherited disorders. Genetic testing and counselling becomes much more precise when you know the gene, where it is, and what it codes for. Unfortunately, gene therapy—delivering the gene into the tissues in which it is defective—has proved difficult, and has been achieved so far in only one, non-renal inherited disorder. However, our understanding of *polycystic kidney disease* is moving very rapidly at the moment in two directions. First, the gene for the commoner (adult, dominant) type of cystic kidneys now called PKD1 has been found, isolated, and its complete structure determined. It codes for a protein important in transport of substances into and out of cells, and this presents obvious possibilities for treatment. This already allows us to make the diagnosis of the condition at birth or even earlier, leaving a good deal of time in which we can learn how to deliver the gene into the kidney. Meanwhile, we have begun to understand how cysts form, and treatments directed at the disordered transport of salts and water into the dilated tubules forming the cysts, and against the messages which promote scarring of the substance of the kidney, are already available in the laboratory. Thus even though we may not be able to reconstruct the defective gene for some years, we may be able to avoid its effects.

Other inherited disorders such as *cystinosis* and *oxalosis* depend upon identifying and localizing the defective gene. This has now been done for both conditions, and the site—but not the nature—of the cystinosis gene is now known. Techniques of gene therapy should be applicable to oxalosis and avoid liver transplantation or an auxiliary liver transplantation, without removal of the patient's own liver. Cystinosis, it seems, can be managed already quite effectively if the condition can be diagnosed early in infancy and treatment begun with one of the cysteamine drugs. New versions of these without the unpleasant smell are now available and under trial.

We already know which gene is disordered in most patients with *Alport's syndrome* but the situation is very complex here because many molecules go to making up the defective basement membranes found in the glomerular filters in this condition. Genetic counselling is obviously now very precise, but of course this knowledge carries with it difficult decisions about what to do with regard to having a family.

In the field of *glomerulonephritis* and the nephrotic syndrome, we have learned an enormous amount in the past decade, but this has not yet translated into treatments available in the clinic. However I believe that this knowledge will result very soon in the rapid entry of more specific treatments for glomerulonephritis during the next 5 years, designed to attack the messengers that promote inflammation and scarring within the filters and substances of the kidney. These have already proved successful in the laboratory, and in some other human immune diseases such as rheumatoid arthritis. The same holds true for *systemic lupus erythematosus.* I hope very much that what has been the standard treatment for these diseases, that is non-specific immunosuppression with toxic medicines such as corticosteroids and cyclophosphamide, will shortly become history; after all, they have been with us almost 50 years now!

In *diabetes* prevention has already achieved a great deal: the proportion of young insulin-dependent diabetics who develop kidney disease and kidney failure has fallen from about one half to about one quarter over the past 30 years as a result of better control of the blood glucose with more frequent insulin injections (see Chapter 9). Diet is a key to preventing diabetes in older people, and the intake of calories in many developed societies is still far too high for good health. We have just found that very tight control of the blood sugar can, as we suspected for a long time, help even more, and the challenge now is to apply this at a practical level in everyday life to the very large number of diabetics potentially at risk. It would make all this much easier if we had ways of detecting those diabetics who are genetically 'programmed' to develop kidney failure right at the beginning of their diabetes, and it looks as though this should be possible again by examining DNA.

It almost goes without saying that in the genesis of *blood vessel disease* smoking is a major and totally avoidable factor. When cigarette smoking is regarded as the addiction it is and treatment offered in addiction clinics, rather than being advertised in most media including television in some countries, then we will have made some progress. Healthy eating again has a role to play and gradually people's ideas of a healthy diet is changing in the direction of less animal fats.

It is little appreciated how much kidney failure is the result of *toxic substances* in the environment, and this undoubtedly accounts for some of the very high incidence of kidney failure in the undeveloped and especially the developing world, in which industry has expanded, but without regard to pollution. Lead is only one of many substances which can damage the kidney and cause kidney failure many years later. A clean environment and better food have already cut the incidence of kidney failure tenfold in the developed world over the past century; let us hope this can be extended to the sprawling masses of industrial cities in the developing world over the next few years.

Slowing the progression of kidney disease

Assuming that the original disease cannot be prevented, what can we hope for in the field of slowing progression? Reduced protein diets have proved to be only poorly effective, or not effective at all, in humans and our mainstay is still early detection and reduction of high blood pressure. One question being debated today is whether lowering the blood pressure to lower but still normal levels in those without high blood pressure might help, especially in those with diabetic kidney disease. New ways of treating blood pressure more smoothly, safely, and effectively are already available in the laboratory, and will make it easier and safer to give treatment to a wider group of patients with mild blood pressure.

Treatment of end-stage kidney failure

What progress can we see in the treatment of people who still develop end-stage kidney failure? Certainly there is little prospect for some years that we will see this happening at much the same rate as now for the next few years in the developed world, or only gradually decreasing.

Dialysis

Dialysis is still performed in much the same way as it was 50 years ago, but using more sophisticated, reliable, and convenient apparatus. After strenuous attempts, no-one now seems interested in making a low-efficiency small artificial kidney which is small enough to wear and which operates continuously. The engineering problems of powering blood through such a tiny device are formidable, but probably not insoluble. Nevertheless, I do not see a useful wearable artificial kidney in the next 5–10 years, although this is probably possible in technical terms already. CAPD has of course reduced the need for such a machine, and it could be argued that we already have such a wearable artificial kidney in the form of the peritoneum! However there are still major problems with CAPD despite a decade's progress. On the one hand new exchange systems result in much less peritonitis, but the blunt fact is that the majority of patients are unable for one reason or another to continue CAPD for more than 5–10 years. Better solutions which are less toxic to the cells within and lining the peritoneum containing glucose polymer are under trial and just coming into widespread use; we must hope they will allow longer use of the peritoneum as an auxiliary kidney.

Transplantation

Given that, for decades to come, people will still go into kidney failure, we will still have a need for transplantation of the kidney as the best treatment for the majority of people in need of treatment for end-stage kidney failure.

Transplantation of solid organs such as the kidney (that is, other than skin and bone marrow) has moved very fast during the 30 years it has been a clinical reality. However in some ways we are still using the technology of the 1960s. On the one hand, we try to find a human donor, either a close relative or someone recently dead who 'matches' the person who needs a kidney in terms of their make-up, in particular their HLA type (see Chapter 8), in an attempt to minimize the gap between them. On the other, having done a transplant, we attempt using chemicals (drugs) to blunt the reaction of the recipient to what his or her immune system perceives as 'foreign' about the graft, at the price of blunting all reactions against foreign antigens, thus exposing the recipient to a considerable increase in infections and a small increase in the number of cancers.

Of course the art of matching and exchange of kidneys has improved enormously over the past 20 years, and we now recognize that better matching improves graft survival of transplants by 10–20%, particularly in the long term (5–20 years). Equally, immunosuppressive drugs have improved, and as well as the traditional corticosteroids (prednisolone) and azathioprine (Imuran) we have had cyclosporine for over a decade, which has reduced almost one half the number of kidneys lost in the first year or so. Several other drugs are just coming into the clinic whose impact has yet to be assessed completely, such as mycophenylate mofetil, which is a relative of azathioprine, tacrolimus (FK 506 Prograf), which acts in a similar way to cyclosporine, sirolimus (rapamycin), which despite its name acts in a different way altogether, and brequinar, a very distant relative of azathioprine. New combinations of these drugs may well improve results, but these do not represent a really new approach—only the refining of what is already in place.

There are two ways in which this should change in the near future. The first advance would be to be capable of inducing a *tolerance* in the recipient to the foreign antigens of the donor kidney. Despite the fact that this has been possible for some years by various routes in experimental animals, we have failed miserably so far in achieving this in human transplantation, although interestingly some living donor kidney recipients seem to become completely tolerant of their relative's graft, and can stop all immunosuppression. Sadly, this never seems to happen spontaneously with cadaver grafts, even when present for many years, and stopping immunosuppressive drugs altogether always leads to rejection in a matter of weeks or months. The memory of the immune system is very, very good, unfortunately for transplantation, which is not surprising when one considers that exposure to an infection such as measles confers almost lifelong immunity against the disease.

I think it likely that within five to ten years we will be able to 're-educate' the host's immune system so that it no longer identifies the differences between the donor kidney and 'self'. This would allow the grafted organ to remain in place indefinitely without any immunosuppressive drugs, whilst the reactions of the body against other foreign antigens, such as those on harmful viruses and germs, would remain intact. Clearly this would be an enormous advantage if it could be achieved.

The second major problem in transplantation is shortage of donor organs, as outlined in Chapter 8. I am not optimistic that any changes in people's attitudes or the laws of the country will make a major impact on the number of cadaver kidneys available for transplantation, although a modest increase of up to 45/million/year kidneys should be possible in all the developed countries not yet operating at this level—which is all but Austria and Norway. However we need almost twice this number to be able to transplant everyone who could benefit from this approach. In the short term, using more living donors (as the USA and Norway already do) could help those countries not exploiting this source, but this rasies all the social and family problems discussed in Chapter 8.

A possible solution to this dilemma, which would be a true revolution in transplantation, is *xenotransplantation*: that is, using organs from other species. There will be those who maintain that use of *any* animal in this way, whether closely related to man or not, as a source of spare parts is unethical. The majority of carnivorous mankind would, however accept that they already exploit animals for food and this new use is, if anything, preferable.

This was tried as long ago as the 1960s, and even with ordinary immuno-suppression, one chimpanzee kidney lasted for nine months. However, to use primates close to mankind (chimpanzees and gorillas) is impossible for several reasons. First, there are the ethical problems of whether we could do this from the point of view of how conscious these highly intelligent animals might be of their fate. Even before we consider this knotty problem, another renders it almost irrelevant. The number of chimpanzees in the whole world is only about 200 000, the number of gorillas tenfold less, and there is no way with a breeding programme that this shortage could be remedied, since primates are long-lived, producing only a single offspring at intervals. Baboons are more attractive from this practical point of view, but differ much more from humans so that the advantage of using a closely related species is lost.

We must therefore look elsewhere in the animal kingdom, and we already know that the further we move from humankind, the bigger the immunological barrier will be which we have to surmount. From numerous points of view pigs are ideal. They are not too large, rapidly produce large litters, have been bred already to be relatively free of infections, and are relatively similar in their genetic make-up, and their kidneys and other organs are very similar in size and function to human organs. The big problem is how to make pig kidneys, hearts, livers, or lungs 'acceptable' to the human immune system. The worry of introducing unknown viruses into the human system remains. Pigs, like humans, carry viruses in their DNA and in their cells, and no-one knows what the effects might be of some of the pig viruses in someone probably receiving immunosuppressive drugs. At the moment, we simply do not know whether this is going to be a major problem, and if so, how great.

Clearly one could do this by manipulating the recipient (human) system so that it did not recognize 'pig' on the cells of the pig kidney or other organ. This would be an even bigger task than re-educating the immune system to accept minor differences from other humans. The other approach is to alter the pig, so that it becomes more 'human'—that is, to alter or eliminate the antigens which humans can recognize when presented with an organ from another species in their circulation.

This task is formidable. If a graft from one species which is 'discordant' that is, not close like a primate kidney is to man, is placed into another species, the recipient treats the graft as a solid lump of foreign bacteria and unleashes an intense immunological attack; within minutes the whole circulation clots solid, the organ turns blue and then black, and is completely destroyed. We know that this starts with antibodies we are all born with, which react with sugar molecules on the surface of the pig cells, which all animals except primates have there. Could we block these antibodies, or stop them from doing harm?

At the time of writing there is intense effort in Europe and the United States to solve this problem. The basic approaches are on the one hand, to 'knock out' genes which code for antigens important in triggering the (xenograft) transplant reaction, or on the other to insert new human genes—short stretches of DNA—which could make the lining of the pig blood vessels seem more human, carried over in the DNA of a yeast. This is done to the single fertilized egg of the pig, which is then replaced in the uterus so that it can mature into a whole animal. Then the animal can be bread from to produce a family of pigs which will have the same altered gene as their mother.

At the moment, it looks likely that it will be possible at least in part, to block or avoid the acute reaction after a xenograft is put in. What would happen then is conjecture; we simply do not know whether humans will recognize the pig equivalent of the HLA tissue antigens, and how strong or weak this reaction will be. The future of an unlimited supply of readily available organs for transplantation depends on the answer to this question. It may even be possible to 'customize' a pig or pigs to suit a single individual, or group of individuals, who have particular HLA tissue types, by inserting sequences within the area of their DNA which codes for their tissue types.

Growing a new kidney

Finally, the possibility of growing whole kidneys in the laboratory from human cells—perhaps the cells of the very person needing treatment—is attractive but immensely complicated. We simply do not know the structure of the template that the DNA carries which tells the mass of cells which are to become a kidney to organize themselves into one. However, in theory it should be possible.

Appendix 1

Commonly used abbreviations in nephrology

A	arterial (used in dialysis) tissue type locus (HLA-A)
ADH	anti-diuretic hormone
AGN	acute glomerulonephritis
ALG/ATG	anti-lymphocyte/anti-thymocyte globulin
APD (cf CCPD)	automated peritoneal dialysis
ARF	acute renal failure
B	tissue type locus (HLA-B)
BUN	blood urea nitrogen
CAPD	continuous ambulatory peritoneal dialysis
CAT scan	computed axial tomographic scan
CCPD	continuous cycling peritoneal dialysis (cf APD)
CMV	cytomegalovirus
CRF	chronic renal failure
DR	tissue type locus (HLA-DR)
EBV	Epstein–Barr (glandular fever) virus
EPO	erythropoietin
ESRD/ESRF	end-stage renal disease/failure
ESWL	extracorporeal shock-wave lithotripsy
GFR	glomerular filtration rate
HD	haemodialysis
HLA	human leukocyte antigen (tissue type)
HSP	Henoch–Schönlein purpura
HUS	haemolytic–uraemic syndrome
IV	intravenous line, injection, infusion
IVU/IVP	intravenous urogram/pyelogram

*K*t/*V*	measure of efficiency of dialysis
MCU	micturating cysto-urethrogram
MLR/MLC	mixed lymphocyte reaction/culture
MRI	magnetic resonance imaging
NMR	nuclear magnetic resonance image (now MRI)
PD	peritoneal dialysis
RBC	red blood cells
RDT	regular dialysis treatment
TX	transplantation
V	venous
WBC	white blood cell

Appendix 2

Organizations concerned with the welfare of kidney patients and information on kidney diseases. This list is by no means complete and further information may be obtained on the internet http://www.md.umich.edu/trans/transweb/support/aakp.Gtml

United Kingdom

The British Kidney Patient Association (BKPA)

President: Mrs Elizabeth Despard Ward OBE Hon. LLD

Oakhanger Place
Bordon, Hants GU35 9JZ

Tel: Bordon (01420) 472021/2
Fax: Bordon (01420) 475831

The BKPA concerns itself with all aspects of provision of care for kidney patients including:

(i) Aid to individual patients. This is normally channelled through the social worker attached to the appropriate Kidney Unit, but individual kidney patients and/or their relatives may become members. Aid may take the form of purchasing necessities, or cash payments for travel, special diets, special equipment, etc.

(ii) Holiday dialysis treatment at a BKPA holiday dialysis centre on the South Coast of England, or on Jersey in the Channel Islands.

(iii) To provide a forum for channelling and exerting local and national pressure on legislators and administrators on matters of concern to kidney patients, especially the level of provision of treatment, availability of donor organs, etc.

(iv) Aid to renal units caring for kidney patients, where such aid will directly benefit patient care. For example, 'pump priming' appointments of social workers or special nurses. Major aid has been given previously to help in the construction or setting up of new treatment facilities.

The BKPA has money earmarked for children and children's needs, as well as a general fund for adult patients.

The BKPA does not raise money for research into kidney disorders.

The National Kidney Federation (NKF)

Chairmen: Frank Howarth and David Poulter
National Coordinator: Margaret Jackson

6 Stanley Street
Worksop S81 7HX

Tel: 01909 487795
Fax: 01909 481723

The National Kidney Federation includes representatives of all the Patients' Associations from each of the individual Kidney Units in the UK. Its aims are to further the interests of patients with kidney disease, to disseminate information, hold meetings, and bring to the attention of local and national politicians issues which affect kidney patients.

National Kidney Research Fund and Kidney Foundation

Chairman: Professor Andrew J. Rees MD FRCP

Director General: Leslie Rout FBIM AMIPR

3 Archers Court
Stukely Road
Huntingdon PE18 6XG
England

Tel: 01480 454 828
Fax: 01480 454 683

These bodies raise money for research into the causes and alleviation of diseases of the kidney in both children and adults, and as such have no direct connection with patient care or aid. On the other hand they are the major funding bodies supporting kidney research into kidney diseases in the UK. They work in concert with other groups, such as the KRUF in Wales.

KRUF

R. Gabe-Wilkinson
14 Park Grove
Cardiff CF1 3BN
Wales
Tel: 01222 388353
Fax: 01222 344130

This body was founded to promote research into, and the care of patients with kidney disease in Wales, but has since become a national organization.

Other national bodies which fund kidney research are:

The Medical Research Council

20 Park Crescent
Regent's Park
London W1N 6DE
Tel: 0171 636 5422
Fax: 0171 436 6179

The Wellcome Trust

183 Euston Road
London NW1 2DT
Tel: 0171 611 8888
Fax: 0171 611 8352

United States of America

National Kidney Foundation Inc.

Executive director: John Davies, CEI
Marketing Director: Ellie Schlam
President (1996): M. Martinez-Maldonado, MD

National office:
30 East Third Street, Suite 1000
New York NY 10016

Tel: 1 800 622 9010/212 889 2210
Fax: 212 689 9261

This is a national organization which has chapters in all states of the union, several in some of the larger states such as California and Texas. A list of addresses and officers can be obtained from the central office.

Its aims are broad, covering a wide range of activities in disseminating information about kidney disease, acting on behalf of those with kidney disorders, coordinating the efforts of those looking after kidney patients, raising money and funding research, and holding clinical and scientific meetings. The NKF has a large amount of informational material on various kidney diseases which is regularly updated and distributed nationwide. In addition many state NKF organizations produce their own material.

American Kidney Fund

Executive director: F.J. Soldavere CAE
President: D. J. Garner CPA

6110 Executive Boulevard, Suite 1010
Rockville MD 20852
USA
Tel: 1 800 639 9299
     (301) 881 3052
Fax: (301) 881 0898

The American Kidney Fund provides direct assistance, including finance, to patients who cannot afford treatments, and is the only national organization in the USA fulfilling this need. It also disseminates information on kidney diseases and kidney failure, and supports local and national meetings on kidney disease. Grants are reviewed and issued quarterly by a Board of Trustees, and cover such items as medicines, travel costs, dialysis costs, and special diets.

American Association of Kidney Patients

President: Joseph D. White
Vice President: Lynn Wasserman
Program manager: Joseph Nadglowski Jr.
Executive Director: Kris Robinson

100 South Ashley Drive
Suite 280
Tampa, Florida 33260
USA

Tel: 1 800 449 2257
    813 223 7099
Fax: 813 223 0001

The AAKP (formerly the NAPHT— National Association for patients on haemodialysis and transplant) has now been in operation for more than 20 years, dedicated to helping patients with kidney disease and their families. There are 20 chapters throughout the USA and a list can be obtained from the central office. The AAKP acts as a spokesperson for kidney patients in local and national political fora, provides information and education about kidney diseases to patients and interested bodies, and organizes national and local meetings for information exchange. A strong feature has been emphasis on disablement and rehabilitation. It has concerned itself with both patient choice and standards of treatment.

National Kidney Patients' Association

President: Perry S. Ecksel
Executive Director: Stuart Kaufer

804 Second St. Pike
Southampton PA 18966
USA

National Kidney and Urologic Diseases Information Clearinghouse

3 Information Way
Bethesda MD 20892-3580
USA

Tel: (301) 654 4415

This has been set up as an aid to the NIDDKD (National Institute of Diabetes Digestive and Kidney Diseases) of the National Institutes of Health (NIH). It aims to provide information to both professionals and patients about, amongst other areas, kidney and urologic diseases, and has a large number of booklets on kidney and urologic problems, as well as providing physicians with information.

Ireland

Irish Kidney Association

c/o Mrs P. Doherty
Chief Executive
Donor House
156 Pembroke Road
Ballsbridge, Dublin 4
Ireland
Tel: 35 31 6689788

Singapore

National Kidney Foundation

Medical director: Dr Hugh Feidhlim Woods
Nursing Director: Ms Anne Flett
Executive secretary: Lynn Ng

Hougang Dialysis Centre
Block 114 Hougang Avenue 1
Unit 01-1298
Singapore 1953
Tel: (65) 287 9893
Fax: (65) 383 0203

Canada

The Kidney Foundation of Canada (La Fondation Canadienne du Rein)

National office:
780–5160 Boulevard Decarie
Montreal, Que H3X 2H9

President: Vivian Doyle-Kelly
Executive Director: Gavin Turley

Tel: 1 800 361 7494
       514 368 4806
Fax: 514 369 2472

The Kidney Foundation of Canada is a national volunteer organization dedicated to improving the health and quality of life of people living with kidney disease. There are individual offices in every province of Canada (three in Ontario), and a list of these can be obtained from the central office. It funds research and related clinical education, provides services for the special needs of individuals living with kidney disease, prepares and circulates literature and information for patients, runs holiday dialysis camps, advocates access to high quality health care, and promotes awareness of and commitment to organ donation.

Australia

Australian Kidney Foundation

This is made up of a series of state-based associations which link together for purposes of national affairs, but operate locally and are based on the different states that make up the Union of Australia. The aims and organization of the different associations is however broadly similar.

Queensland Renal Association Inc.

GPO Box 3093
Brisbane QLD 4001
Queensland

Tel: 07 832 2520
Fax: 07 832 3453

New South Wales Kidney Foundation

Ground floor, 161 Clarence Street
Sydney 2000 NSW

Tel: 02 299 4455
Fax. 02 299 7582

Victoria Kidney Foundation

Suite 207, 620 St Kilda Road
Melbourne, Victoria 3004

Tel: 03 525 1515
Fax: 03 521 1958

South Australia

1st Floor, 82 Melbourne Street
North Adelaide, SA 5006

Tel: 08 267 4555
Fax: 08 267 4450

Western Australia

Ground floor, 220 St George's Terrace
Perth, WA 6000

Tel: 09 322 1354
Fax: 09 481 3707

Tasmania

GPO Box 61
Hobart, Tasmania 7001

Tel: 002 313 053
Fax: 002 233 506

Northern Territory

Room 4, Cauarina Plaza
Casuarina, NT 0810

Tel: 089 454 047

There are also one or two other organizations in Australia concerned with renal patients:

Dialysis and Transplant Association (DATA Inc.)

PO Box 125
Blackburn, Victoria 3130

Renal and pancreas transplants

RAPT PO Box 414
Toongabbie, NSW 2146

Dialysis and Renal Transplant Association of Western Australia

3 Melrose Street
Rossmoyne, WA 6148

New Zealand

Auckland District Kidney Association Inc.
PO Box 97026
South Auckland Mail Centre
Manukau City
New Zealand

Aid and information for patients with particular diseases:

Diabetes mellitus

The British Diabetic Association

President: Professor Harry Keen

10 Queen Anne Street
London W1M 9LD
England
Tel: 0171 323 1531
Fax: 0171 637 3644

The BDA provides support and information for all diabetics, including those
with kidney problems. They have published material for diabetics with kidney
disease, including *Living with kidney disease and diabetes*.

The American Diabetes Association

President: Kathleen Wishner
Director of International Relations: Linda Cann

1660 Duke Street
Alexandria VA 22314
USA

Tel: 1-800-232-3472
    (703) 549 1500
Fax: (703) 683 1839

This concerns itself with a wide range of issues concerning diabetics, including those with renal disease: diagnosis, information, benefits, political issues.

Polycystic kidney disease

Polycystic Kidney Research Foundation

922 Walnut, Suite 411
Kansas City, MO 64106-1826

Tel: 1-800 753 2873

The PK Research Foundation is a nationwide organization for those suffering from all forms of polycystic kidney disease, adult dominantly inherited PKD and childhood recessively inherited PKD in particular, and was founded in 1992. There are groups active in many states and a list of addresses can be obtained from the central office. The Foundation provides support and contacts for those with PKD and their families, prepares information on cystic disease, raises funds for research, and donates grants for research into all forms of cystic disease.

A number of British patients and families are associated with this since there is no comparable British organization.

Cystinosis and oxalosis

Research Trust for Metabolic Disease in Children

Golden Gates Lodge
Weston Road
Crewe CW1 1XN
England

Tel: 01270 250221

This is an 'umbrella' organization and deals with children and families with numerous inherited disorders, including those affecting the kidney.

Cystinosis Foundation

The Cystinosis Foundation Inc.
1212 Broadway, Suite 830
Oakland Ca 94612
USA
Tel: 00 1 510 235 1052

This group has members all over, as well as outside the USA and helps patients and families affected by cystinosis.

Disorders of purine metabolism (xanthinuria, 2-8 DHAuria, HPRT deficiency (Lesch–Nyhan Syndrome), familial juvenile hyperuricaemic nephopathy (FJHN-familial gout)

Purine Metabolic Patients Association (PUMPA)

E. Elspeth Parkes
Honorary Secretary
Purine Metabolic Patients Association
43 Ennismore Gardens
London SW7 1AW
England

This group provides information and aid for patients and their families suffering from the various rare inherited disorders of purine metabolism, including those affecting the kidney.
   They also raise money to support research into the area.

Systemic lupus erythematosus

United Kingdom

Arthritis Care

Olivia Hanscombe
Information
Lupus Group Arthritis Care
18 Stephenson Way
London NW1 2HD

Arthritis care is a group concerned with all forms of arthritis, including systemic lupus.

Lupus UK

51 North Street
Romford, Essex RM1 1BA

Tel: 01708 731251
Fax: 01708 731252

This group provides support and advice for patients with lupus. It also helps raise research funds for the lupus clinic at St Thomas' Hospital, London SE1.

USA

Lupus Foundation of America

4 Research Place, Suite 180
Rockville, MD 20850-3226
USA

Tel: 301 670 9292
Fax: 301 670 9486

The purpose of the Lupus Foundation is to assist their local chapters in their efforts to provide supportive services to individuals living with lupus, to educate the public about lupus, and to support research into the cause and cure of lupus. Volunteers, through an extensive network of over 500 constituent chapters, branches, support groups and International Associated groups, provide the majority of services which link the Lupus Foundation the thousands of lupus patients and their families.

Information resources including brochures and articles are available on request for people seeking an understanding of lupus. The information encompasses many aspects of lupus, including kidney disease, steroids, and cytotoxic medications.

Wegener's granulomatosis

Stuart Strange Trust

Chairman: Mrs S. Fisher
14 Elthorne Way
Newport Pagnall
Bucks MK16 0JH
England
Tel: 0908 611450

This trust promotes knowledge of Wegener's granulomatosis and provides information and support to patients with the disease, and their families.

Haemolytic-uraemic syndrome

Lois Joy Galler Foundation
for Hemolytic Uremic Syndrome, Inc.

President: Robert C. Galler
Vice President: Professor Bernard S. Kaplan MD

753 Walt Whitman Road
Melville, NY 11747
Tel: (516) 673 3017
Fax: (516) 673 3025

This foundation was started by her parents in memory of Lois Joy, who died of HUS. It aims to raise public awareness of HUS, provide information and support for families of parents with the condition, and support research into the disease.

Index

Bold type indicates the main section where there are several entries

obstructions (*cont.*)
  pain from 20
  in people with paraplegia 163
  prostate gland enlargement 17, 45-8
  of ureter 20, 44-8
  of urethra 45 (*Fig.*), 46, 49, *Plate 5*
  see also stones
oedema (swelling) **19-21**, 54-6, 71, *Plate 1*
OKT3 141, 142
operations
  for prostate problems 47
  for stones 47
  for transplantation 127, 137-40, 167
oscillometry 35
osteomalacia 13, 72
osteoporosis after transplantation 147
outcome
  dialysis techniques 180 (*Fig.*)
  glomerulonephritis 56
  transplantation 123-5, 128, 135,
    149-55, 173, 175, 194 (*Fig.*)
  see also survival
oxalosis (hyperoxaluria) 30, 46, **64-5**
  children 64-5, 164
  future understanding of 197
  research in 215
oxprenolol (Trasicor) 40 (*Box*)

pain 20
  back 97, 117
  bone 104
  chest 71, 97
  colicky (renal/ureteric colic) 20
  headache 33
  hip 72, 148
  kidney donation operation 137
  kidney stones 46
  leg 159
  from obstructions 20
  on passing urine 20
  pelvic 72
  in peritonitis 116
  in polycystic disease 58
  after shingles 146
  in sickle-cell disease 67
  in transplantation 140
pain killers, *see* analgesics
pallor 21, 71, 76
  see also anaemia
pancreas transplant in diabetes 161-2
panel reactivity 125 (*Box*)
papilla of kidney 7 (*Fig.*)

papillary necrosis 49, 67
papillomavirus 146
paraplegia and kidney failure 162-4
parathyroid glands and hormone (PTH) 73,
    75, 80, 104, 115
parental donation to children 127, 167
patients' associations 83, 100, 105, 206-18
PD cycler machine 114
pelvic-ureteric junction (PUJ) obstruction
    45 (*Fig.*)
pelvis of kidney 7 (*Fig.*), 8, *Plate 4*, *Plate 7*
  obstruction of 45 (*Fig.*), 46, 49
penicillamine 46
pericarditis 71, 74
peritoneal dialysis
  automated (APD), *see* automated
      peritoneal dialysis
  continuous ambulatory (CAPD), *see* CAPD
  continuous cycling (CCPD), *see*
      automated peritoneal dialysis
  machine, *see* automated peritoneal dialysis
peritoneum 108
  peritonitis 109, 112, **115-16**
personality changes after transplantation
    147
phenacetin 49, 50
phosphate (phosphorus) 73, 75, 76
  binding of 80, 100, 104, 117, 165
  in children 165
  during dialysis 100-1, 115, 117, 118
  after transplantation 144
phosphocysteamine 52
'piggyback' grafts 153
pigs, transplantation from xii, 136, 202-3
pissoirs of Paris 16
pituitary gland 11 (*Fig.*)
plasma transfusion in HUS 66
pneumonia 74
political issues 178, 179, 190
polyangiitis 51-2
polyarteritis (vasculitis) 51-2
polycystic kidney disease (PKD) 30 (*Table*),
    57-63, *Plate 12*
  adult form 58, 59 (*Fig.*), 61-2
  childhood form 30 (*Table*), 61, 64
  complications of 63
  future understanding of 197
  impact on family 62-3
  and transplantation 64, 137
Polycystic Kidney Research Foundation 215
potassium
  during dialysis 102, 118, 119
  in diet 80